HEALTHY LIVING JOURNAL

TRACK YOUR HEALTHY EATING AND LIVING HABITS
FOR IMPROVED HEALTH AND WELL-BEING

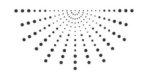

SUSAN U. NEAL

CHRISTIAN INDIE
PUBLISHING

Editor: Janis Whipple

Cover Design: Angie Alaya

Printed in the United States of America

ISBN: 978-0-997-76369-0

CONTENTS

Disclaimer   vii
Journal Belongs to   xi

1. Journal Benefits   1
2. How to Use This Journal   2
3. Healthy Living Goals   5
4. Measurements   8
5. Gratitude Log   10
6. Victory Log   12
7. Blank Log   14
8. Temptation/Struggle Log   15
9. Binge Eating Tracker   17
10. Issue Tracker   19
11. New Healthy Living Habits Log   21
12. Blank Tracker   23
13. Water Tracker   24
14. Steps Tracker   27
15. Fitness Tracker   32
16. Weekly Entry Instructions   35
17. Daily Food Journal Instructions   37

Part I
WEEK 1
Menu Plan   41
Well-Being Chart   45
1. Day 1: Introduction   49
2. Day 2: Decide to Improve Your Health   52
3. Day 3: Healthy Eating Guidelines   55
4. Day 4: How Different Foods Affect Your Body   59
5. Day 5: Menu Planning   62
6. Day 6: Journal Time   65
7. Day 7: Sabbath Reflections   67

Part II
WEEK 2
Menu Plan   71
Well-Being Chart   75
8. Day 8: Acquire Knowledge   77
9. Day 9: Food Addiction   79
10. Day 10: Candida   83
11. Day 11: Seven-Step Plan   86
12. Day 12: Foods to Eliminate   89
13. Day 13: Journal Time   92
14. Day 14: Sabbath Reflections   94

Part III
WEEK 3
Menu Plan   99
Well-Being Chart   103
15. Day 15: Accountability/Prayer Partner   105
16. Day 16: Temptation and the Sword of the Spirit   108
17. Day 17: Prayer   112
18. Day 18: Meditating with God   115
19. Day 19: Five-Steps to Freedom from Addiction   118
20. Day 20: Journal Time   122
21. Day 21: Sabbath Reflections   124

Part IV
WEEK 4
Menu Plan   129
Well-Being Chart   133
22. Day 22: Emotional Issues with Food   135
23. Day 23: Clean Out Your Emotions   140
24. Day 24: Boredom/Stress Eating   143
25. Day 25: Binging   146
26. Day 26: Fight Food Temptation   149
27. Day 27: Journal Time   152
28. Day 28: Sabbath Reflections   154

Part V
WEEK 5
Menu Plan   159

Well-Being Chart   163

29. Day 29: Digestive Issues   165
30. Day 30: Foods That Cause Inflammation   167
31. Day 31: Food Substitutes   170
32. Day 32: Tips for a Healthier Lifestyle   173
33. Day 33: 80/20 Percent Rule   176
34. Day 34: Journal Time   179
35. Day 35: Sabbath Reflections   181

Part VI
WEEK 6

Menu Plan   185
Well-Being Chart   189

36. Day 36: Exercise   191
37. Day 37: Practice Gratitude   194
38. Day 38: Fruit of the Spirit: Self-Control   197
39. Day 39: Plan for the Pitfalls   201
40. Day 40: Improve Your Health   204
41. Day 41: Journal Time   207
42. Day 42: Sabbath Reflections   209

Appendix 1: Food Addiction Battle Strategies   211
Appendix 2: My Battle Strategies Plan   213
Appendix 3: Healthy Food Options   215
Notes   219
About the Author   221
Other Products by Susan Neal   225

DISCLAIMER

Medical Disclaimer: This book offers health and nutritional information, which is for educational purposes only. The information provided in this book is designed to help individuals make informed decisions about their health; it is intended to supplement, not replace, the professional medical advice, diagnosis, or treatment of health conditions from a trained medical professional. Please consult your physician or healthcare provider before beginning or changing any health or eating habits to make sure that it is appropriate for you. If you have any concerns or questions about your health, you should always ask a physician or other healthcare provider. Please do not disregard, avoid, or delay obtaining medical or health-related advice from your healthcare professional because of something you may have read in this book. The author and publisher assume no responsibility for any injury that may result from changing your health or eating habits.

Disclaimer and Terms of Use: Every effort has been made to ensure the information in this book is accurate and complete. However, the author and publisher do not warrant the accuracy or completeness of the material, text, and graphics contained in this book. The author and publisher do not hold any responsibility for

This book is dedicated to:

Edie Melson, for inspiring me to make this a journal with charts,
and
my daughter Shelby, for her encouragement, feedback, and help with
designing the charts.

JOURNAL BELONGS TO

This is the day that the LORD has made;
let us rejoice and be glad in it.
Psalm 118:24 (ESV)

This journal belongs to

_____

1

JOURNAL BENEFITS

Have you tried to decrease your weight or improve your health without success? Or maybe you lost the weight, but it came right back. This journal will help you make lifelong changes so you can reclaim the abundant life Jesus wants you to experience, not a life filled with disease and poor health.

This journal may help you:

- feel and look better
- increase energy
- grow in faith and grace
- sharpen clarity of mind
- harness God's strength to make changes
- become aware of negative food habits
- identify and eliminate behaviors that sabotage your health
- lose weight naturally without a fad diet or buying prepared meals and supplements

I hope you take this journey to improve your well-being.

HOW TO USE THIS JOURNAL

The *Healthy Living Journal* can be used independently or along with *7 Steps to Get Off Sugar and Carbohydrates*. Each day's entry helps you record daily water intake, exercise, and corresponding moods and energy. Recording your daily food consumption provides an opportunity to learn how food affects your health. When you discover negative health patterns you can change.

The first few logs and charts in this journal (located in the front of the book) will be used intermittently to track:

- Gratitude Log—things you are grateful for
- Victory Log—when you succeed in overcoming a food temptation, issue, or other pertinent item
- Blank Log—whatever you want
- Temptation/Struggle Log—things that tempt you to overeat and struggle with food
- Binge Eating Tracker—each time you binge and its corresponding effects
- Issue Tracker—undesirable health symptoms

- New Healthy Living Habits Log—each positive habit you want to incorporate into your life
- Blank Tracker—whatever you want

The Blank Log and Tracker are left blank for you to track you own specific issues.

The next three charts should be completed on a daily basis:

- Water Tracker
- Steps Tracker
- Fitness Tracker

The journal is divided into six weeks. Each week contains two charts that should be completed on a daily basis:

- Well-Being Chart
- Daily Food Journal

Color the corresponding boxes in the Well-Being Chart red when you experience negative symptoms and green when you experience positive symptoms. This will help you figure out what type of food makes your body function well or poorly.

Devotions and educational snippets are provided daily. Learn about food addiction, Candida infection of the gut, and healthy eating guidelines from these daily entries. As you gain knowledge, you will learn how to improve your health and weight. You will also journal and spend time with God. You are a child of God and deserve the most life has to offer you. Choose to take the time needed to improve your health; your body will thank you.

If you would like to dive deeper, a corresponding course, 7 Steps to Reclaim Your Health and Optimal Weight is available at Susan-UNeal.com/courses/7-steps-to-get-off-sugar-and-carbs-course. This course shows you how to use this book and *7 steps to Get Off Sugar and Carbohydrates* to meet your healthy living goals.

3
HEALTHY LIVING GOALS

Document the specific goals you would like to achieve.

Health

1.

2.

3.

Eating Habits

1.

2.

3.

Meal Planning

1.

2.

3.

Physical Activity

1.

2.

3.

Stress Relief

1.

2.

3.

Weight

1.

2.

3.

Sleep

1.

2.

3.

GOALS
ONE DAY AT A TIME
ONE MEAL AT A TIME
ONE WORKOUT AT A TIME

There is a time for everything,
and a season for every activity under the heavens.
Ecclesiastes 3:1 (NIV)

4

MEASUREMENTS

Document the specific goals you would like to achieve in reference to your measurements. However, seek progress not perfection.

1.

2.

3.

4.

5.

Measurements	Start Date	End Date
Upper Arms		
Chest		
Waist		
Hips		
Thighs		
Calves		
Weight		

SEEK PROGRESS
NOT PERFECTION

5

GRATITUDE LOG

Record things you are grateful for.

1.

2.

3.

4.

5.

6.

. . .

7.

8.

9.

10.

11.

12.

13.

14.

15.

Sing psalms and hymns and spiritual songs to God with thankful
hearts.
Colossians 3:16

VICTORY LOG

Record any victory you achieved, no matter how small it may be.

1.

2.

3.

4.

5.

6.

. . .

7.

8.

9.

10.

11.

12.

13.

14.

15.

The Lord is my strength and my song; he has given me **victory**. This
is my God, and I will praise him!
Exodus 15:2

7

BLANK LOG

TEMPTATION/STRUGGLE LOG

Determine if there is a pattern to your struggles by documenting the temptation here.

1.

2.

3.

4.

5.

6.

. . .

7.

8.

9.

10.

11.

12.

13.

14.

15.

And don't let us yield to **temptation**, but rescue us from the evil one.
Matthew 6:13

BINGE EATING TRACKER

Every time you binge, record the incident in the following Binge Eating Tracker chart. The items on the right side of the of the chart are for tracking your symptoms after you overate. Add a Y for yes and N for no for those items. Recognize if there is a correlation between energy level, mental clarity, and mood after binging. Also, note whether you experienced any digestive discomfort.

Determine your feelings before you binged and what temptation led you down that path. Did something trigger the episode? Figure out your trigger and record it in the Temptation/Struggle Log. After a while you may find a pattern—the same sort of situation or item tempts you. When you understand what entices you, you can learn to avoid it.

After binging, ask God to forgive you and help you not to binge again. Record your experience in the blank pages of the sixth or seventh day of each week's journal. These page are left blank to allow space for you to journal your thoughts and concerns.

If you record every incident of overeating in the following Binge Eating Tracker you will reduce the number of times you binge. Retraining your mind is like disciplining a child; consistency is vital to transformation. Ask God to help you along the way and he will.

Day	Time	Food	Qty.	Trigger /Why	Digestive Issue?	Low Energy Level?	Poor Mental Clarity?	Bad Mood?

Let us strip off every weight that slows us down, especially the sin that
so easily trips us up. And let us run with endurance the race God has
set before us.
Hebrews 12:1

ISSUE TRACKER

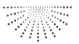

Whether you have a digestive issue or difficulty sleeping (it doesn't matter what the problem is), use this page to track when the issue occurs and what you ate up to twelve hours prior to the problem, so you can identify the culprit (example: foods containing MSG may disturb sleep or cause allergies).

DATE / PROBLEM / FOOD CONSUMED WITHIN 12 HRS

1.

2.

3.

4.

. . .

5.

6.

7.

8.

9.

10.

11.

12.

13.

14.

15.

Dear friend, I hope all is well with you and that you are as healthy in
body as you are strong in spirit.
3 John 2

NEW HEALTHY LIVING HABITS LOG

What new habits would you like to embrace?

1.

2.

3.

4.

5.

6.

. . .

7.

8.

9.

10.

11.

12.

13.

14.

15.

In everything you do, put God first, and he will direct you and crown
your efforts with success.
Proverbs 3:6 (TLB)

12
BLANK TRACKER

WATER TRACKER

It is essential to stay hydrated. However, we shouldn't appease our thirst with sugar-sweetened beverages because they fog the mind. Instead, we should drink the fluid God gave us—water. Our bodies desperately need water to flush out toxins and prevent dehydration.

The human body is comprised of 75 percent water, and we can't survive for more than a few days without it. Some people think drinking tea, juice, soda, or other drinks will hydrate their body, but they won't. In fact, caffeinated beverages are a diuretic, which cause you to urinate more frequently and lose fluids.

Water requirements depend upon your size. Various sources recommend: "Drink half your weight in ounces every day." Using this formula, a 130-pound person should drink eight glasses of water per day. (130/2 = 65 ounces; 65/8 ounces (1 cup) = 8 glasses.) Drink water in between meals, on an empty stomach, and up to fifteen minutes before you eat.

Day	Intake
1	◊◊◊◊◊◊◊◊◊◊
2	◊◊◊◊◊◊◊◊◊◊
3	◊◊◊◊◊◊◊◊◊◊
4	◊◊◊◊◊◊◊◊◊◊
5	◊◊◊◊◊◊◊◊◊◊
6	◊◊◊◊◊◊◊◊◊◊
7	◊◊◊◊◊◊◊◊◊◊
8	◊◊◊◊◊◊◊◊◊◊
9	◊◊◊◊◊◊◊◊◊◊
10	◊◊◊◊◊◊◊◊◊◊
11	◊◊◊◊◊◊◊◊◊◊
12	◊◊◊◊◊◊◊◊◊◊
13	◊◊◊◊◊◊◊◊◊◊
14	◊◊◊◊◊◊◊◊◊◊
15	◊◊◊◊◊◊◊◊◊◊
16	◊◊◊◊◊◊◊◊◊◊
17	◊◊◊◊◊◊◊◊◊◊
18	◊◊◊◊◊◊◊◊◊◊
19	◊◊◊◊◊◊◊◊◊◊
20	◊◊◊◊◊◊◊◊◊◊
21	◊◊◊◊◊◊◊◊◊◊

"For the Scriptures declare that rivers of living water shall flow from the inmost being of anyone who believes in me."
John 7:38 (TLB)

Day	Intake
22	〇〇〇〇〇〇〇〇
23	〇〇〇〇〇〇〇〇
24	〇〇〇〇〇〇〇〇
25	〇〇〇〇〇〇〇〇
26	〇〇〇〇〇〇〇〇
27	〇〇〇〇〇〇〇〇
28	〇〇〇〇〇〇〇〇
29	〇〇〇〇〇〇〇〇
30	〇〇〇〇〇〇〇〇
31	〇〇〇〇〇〇〇〇
32	〇〇〇〇〇〇〇〇
33	〇〇〇〇〇〇〇〇
34	〇〇〇〇〇〇〇〇
35	〇〇〇〇〇〇〇〇
36	〇〇〇〇〇〇〇〇
37	〇〇〇〇〇〇〇〇
38	〇〇〇〇〇〇〇〇
39	〇〇〇〇〇〇〇〇
40	〇〇〇〇〇〇〇〇
41	〇〇〇〇〇〇〇〇
42	〇〇〇〇〇〇〇〇

STEPS TRACKER

Fitbits, Apple watches, and smartphones provide the wearer with the number of steps that they take each day. Technology is amazing, isn't it? But wearing all those devices can't make us get up and move. However, when you eat well, you feel better and this increase in energy can get you moving!

Every day record the number of steps you take either by coloring the boxes to notate the level of your steps or write the number of steps in the corresponding box.

After a week a two of eating well, you will get a new sense of energy. So get out there and walk, even if it is only down the block and back.

	Day 1	Day 2	Day 3	Day 4	Day 5	Day 6	Day 7	Day 8	Day 9	Day 10
10k										
9k										
8k										
8k										
7k										
6k										
5k										
4k										
3k										
2k										
1k										

The steps of good men are directed by the Lord. He delights in each
step they take.
Psalm 37:23 (TLB)

	Day 11	Day 12	Day 13	Day 14	Day 15	Day 16	Day 17	Day 18	Day 19	Day 20	Day 21
10k											
9k											
8k											
8k											
7k											
6k											
5k											
4k											
3k											
2k											
1k											

	Day 22	Day 23	Day 24	Day 25	Day 26	Day 27	Day 28	Day 29	Day 30	Day 31
10k										
9k										
8k										
8k										
7k										
6k										
5k										
4k										
3k										
2k										
1k										

10k											
9k											
8k											
8k											
7k											
6k											
5k											
4k											
3k											
2k											
1k											
	Day 32	Day 33	Day 34	Day 35	Day 36	Day 37	Day 38	Day 39	Day 40	Day 41	Day 42

FITNESS TRACKER

Physical exercise is not only beneficial for the body, but it also enhances brain function. Yes, it makes your brain work better, and it releases endorphins in the brain that improve your mood and sense of well-being. Exercising, a positive coping strategy for dealing with stress, burns off adrenaline and improves sleep. Regular physical activity helps to prevent chronic diseases such as diabetes, obesity, depression, cancer, and heart disease.

Varying the types of fitness activity that you perform is beneficial. In the winter, I walk a couple of miles a week. But in the summer, I swim twenty laps in my pool twice a week. Bicycling is an excellent form of exercise to perform when it is hot outside.

I also have a vegetable garden and fruit orchard. I consider gardening and yard work a rigorous form of physical activity. You don't have to go to the gym to expend calories; you could just vacuum and mop the whole house. Therefore, I listed several different activities that I consider forms of fitness training.

Record the number of minutes you perform each activity on the following charts.

Day	Cardio	Strength	Group Fitness	Cleaning	Gardening
1					
2					
3					
4					
5					
6					
7					
8					
9					
10					
11					
12					
13					
14					
15					
16					
17					
18					
19					
20					
21					

And let us run with perseverance the race marked out for us, fixing
our eyes on Jesus, the pioneer and perfecter of faith.
Hebrews 12:1-2 (NIV)

Day	Cardio	Strength	Group Fitness	Cleaning	Gardening
22					
23					
24					
25					
26					
27					
28					
29					
30					
31					
32					
33					
34					
35					
36					
37					
38					
39					
40					
41					
42					

1 6

WEEKLY ENTRY INSTRUCTIONS

The first five days of each week include a devotion or educational snippet. However, the sixth and seventh days (Journal Time and Sabbath Reflections) are left blank to allow space for you to journal your thoughts, feelings, desires, and concerns.

Be sure to record daily information in the weekly Well-Being Chart and tracker tables for water, steps, and fitness. In addition, complete a Daily Food Journal provided at the end of each day's devotion.

As you experience:

- temptations—record this in the Temptation/Struggle log
- undesirable health issues—track these symptoms in the Issue Tracker
- binge—document the incident in the Binge Eating Tracker
- gratitude or victory—note this in the appropriate log
- new positive habits—record them in the New Healthy Living Habits Log
- defeat over temptation—write how you succeeded in

overcoming spiritually in Appendix 2: My Battle Strategies Plan

- other items not listed—track them in the Blank Log and Tracker

These logs and charts are at the beginning of this journal and the appendices in the back. Several pages are left blank for you to create your own log or tracker page.

Try not to be overwhelmed by the amount of entries as you begin this journal. Completing the process will only take a few minutes here and there each day, and the benefits of journaling will outweigh the time required.

DAILY FOOD JOURNAL
INSTRUCTIONS

This daily journal will appear after every day's devotion, so you understand how your food intake affects your overall well-being. Take the time each day to complete the chart so you can have a full picture of your journey to health and abundance.

The last three items at the bottom of the chart correspond to your symptoms after you ate. Add a Y for yes and N for no for those items. Recognize if there is a correlation between energy level, mental clarity, and mood after eating. Also, note whether you experienced any digestive discomfort.

After-Dinner Snack

Do not eat anything three hours before going to bed, and fast for twelve hours each night (from dinner until breakfast). This recommendation is for brain health, to prevent dementia and Alzheimer's. A clinical study that showed significant improvement in these diseases of the brain recommends these two interventions to reduce insulin levels.[2] Therefore, if you eat dinner at 7 p.m. and go to bed at 10 p.m., you should not eat a snack after dinner.

	Breakfast	Lunch	Snack	Dinner
Food				
Time				
Three Hours Since Last Meal?				
Hungry?				
Feel an Emotion? Describe:				
Satisfied or Stuffed				
Digestive Issue?				
Poor Mental Clarity?				
Bad Mood?				

PART I
WEEK 1

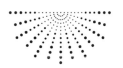

MENU PLAN

Planning my weekly menu takes about an hour, and I usually do this on Sunday. I list what I plan to cook for breakfast, lunch, dinner, and snack for every day of the week. As I choose a recipe, I put the ingredients I need on my corresponding grocery list.

After you create your menu and grocery list (subscribe to Susan-UNeal.com/healthy-living-blog for menus and lists), hit the grocery store or local farmer's market. Once your groceries are put away it is time to start cooking healthy homemade meals. Your body will appreciate your planning and food preparation, and being prepared will keep you from making unhealthy impulsive choices when you grocery shop.

Use the following chart to plan your weekly menu.

Meal	Monday	Tuesday
Breakfast		
Lunch		
Snack		
Dinner		

Meal	Wednesday	Thursday
Breakfast		
Lunch		
Snack		
Dinner		

Be sure to take the time needed each week to plan your menu. If you do, you will have healthy foods on hand and that will decrease the possibility of eating unhealthy meals and snacks.

Meal	Friday	Saturday
Breakfast		
Lunch		
Snack		
Dinner		

Meal	Sunday
Breakfast	
Lunch	
Snack	
Dinner	

WELL-BEING CHART

Determine how habits affect your well-being. Record the number of hours you slept and add a Y for yes and N for no for the other items tracked below. Recognize if there is a correlation between your energy level and mood with the consumption of unhealthy foods.

If you pay attention to your body and how it reacts to different types of food, you can figure out what items to eliminate from your diet. For me, it is anything with a high sugar content. I feel my body surge when I experience a sugar high; then it crashes as my blood-sugar level plummets. Afterward, I feel wiped out and devoid of energy. Unfortunately, the next day I suffer from brain fog and low energy.

When you figure out what food causes your body to react poorly, then you can avoid the food culprit. This is the puzzle you need to figure out. Through using this journal you will put the puzzle together.

Days	1	2	3	4	5	6	7
Hours of Sleep							
Ate Unhealthy Foods: List the foods							
Binged							
Low Energy Level							
Brain Fog							
Bad Mood							
Anxiety							
Irritable							
Digestive Issues							
Physical Activity							
Probiotics							
Spent Time w/ God							

Restful sleep is an essential component of a person's well-being. At least eight hours of sleep per night is recommended for optimal brain health and to prevent dementia and Alzheimer's.[1] These diseases of the brain are on the rise. Most everyone has a loved one or knows someone who suffers from one of these diseases. Your sleep and diet affect your brain. If you slept less than eight hours or consumed unhealthy foods, color the box red in the Well-Being Chart. If you experience a day with high energy and clarity of mind color the corresponding boxes green.

Many of the symptoms listed in the Well-Being Chart (energy, brain fog, mood, anxiety, irritability, digestive issues) are caused by the foods you consume. Recently, I noticed that home-made chocolate-chip cookies made with almond flour and maple syrup, although healthier, still made me irritable and less tolerant. My family does not deserve to be treated in an ill-tempered manner. Once I recognized the culprit, by journaling what I ate, I stopped snacking on the cookies.

Spending time with God can also affect your temperament. Most mornings I try to spend fifteen minutes of quiet, meditative time with the Lord. Getting connected with the Creator of the universe and feeling his presence in my life gives me a better sense of well-being. Asking for his help to maintain a healthy eating pattern gives me newfound strength.

Each week you will be provided with a new Well-Being Chart to complete on a daily basis. At the end of each week review your Daily Food Journal and compare it with your Well-Being Chart to determine how you did food wise along with the corresponding symptoms. When you color boxes red (negative symptoms) and green (positive symptoms) it is easier to figure out what type of food makes your body function well and what doesn't. When you find a food culprit, eliminate it from your diet.

1

DAY 1: INTRODUCTION

During the next six weeks, commit to spending a few minutes each day recording what you ate and drank and how your body reacted to those foods. Food issues you didn't know you had will become apparent because you can identify which items you ate that made you feel less than your best. For example, if I eat something that raises my blood sugar, the next day I experience brain fog and lethargy. How do you feel the day after consuming food with high sugar content? Write it down, and you will find out.

Each week's Daily Food Journal and Well-Being Chart will take you through what you should record. Tracking this information is important for your physical health, yet one of the most valuable components of journaling is recording what takes place in the mind. Understanding the emotional and spiritual implications you may have with food is essential to improving your lifestyle.

If you binge, what happens to your body? Write it down in the Binge Eating Log. Just as it is important to determine the nutritional content of food, it is vital to figure out the strongholds in your mind. A stronghold is something you turn to instead of God. Understanding your thoughts about food is necessary to determine the root cause of a dysfunctional food habit.

Recording thoughts, feelings, struggles, and victories has a powerful effect. Journaling also creates personal accountability. The more you journal, the more easily you'll recognize when you are eating out of emotion or for the wrong reason. You may determine what helped you overcome a struggle. Journaling provides clarity of thoughts, feelings, and desires.

If you need more guidance, I created the course, 7 Steps to Reclaim Your Health and Optimal Weight (SusanUNeal.com/courses/7-steps-to-get-off-sugar-and-carbs-course). This course will help you figure out and resolve the root cause of your inappropriate eating habits. One solved, taming your appetite is much easier. I show you how you can change your eating habits once and for all.

Are you living life to its fullness? Is your health or weight impeding you from embracing a healthy, abundant life? You are about to embark on the bountiful life Jesus has in store for you!

"The thief's purpose is to steal, kill and destroy. My purpose is to give life in all its fullness."

John 10:10 (TLB)

Father,

As I begin this journey to improve my health, help me find the time and motivation to record my thoughts and habits in this journal. Please guide me to reawaken the youth and vitality of the glorious body you gave me. Help me understand how different foods affect my body, so I can know if a specific food is harming me. Thank you in advance for helping me and answering my prayers. In Jesus's name. Amen.

	Breakfast	Lunch	Snack	Dinner
Food				
Time				
Three Hours Since Last Meal?				
Hungry?				
Feel an Emotion? Describe:				
Satisfied or Stuffed				
Digestive Issue?				
Poor Mental Clarity?				
Bad Mood?				

2

DAY 2: DECIDE TO IMPROVE YOUR HEALTH

I am delighted that you decided to reclaim your health. No one can force you to change; it has to be an internal motivation. Whether you are experiencing health issues, carrying excessive weight, or want to get your energy back, I am glad you are taking control of your well-being.

Through recording the information included in this journal, you will begin to solve a puzzle, one you couldn't figure out on your own. Each day you will discover a new piece of the puzzle as you understand what you need to do to improve your health. For example, you may not have been drinking enough water, so you experienced constipation. Or you drank half of your daily calories in a Starbucks Frappuccino, and this caused brain fog and fatigue.

As you uncover each new puzzle piece, you will discover how to make your body feel good again. As your energy improves, you will be motivated to go for a walk or attend a social event. Jesus wants you to live life in all its fullness, not in a worn-out, sick body. So let's get going and find out why you are experiencing ill health or excessive weight. Decide to enrich your lifestyle and record each day's information in this journal, so your health will improve.

Deciding is the first step to transformation. Begin by asking God to make you willing to change. Once you are willing, write down the changes you will make, and commit to them before the Lord. Include the measurable goals you would like to achieve in the Healthy Living Goals section at the beginning of this journal. Ask God to help you and place your success in his loving arms.

Write your commitment below:

_____

_____

_____

_____

Now state in a firm voice (speak out loud) the commitment you just made to God.

Crowds of sick people—blind, lame, or paralyzed—lay on the porches. One of the men lying there had been sick for thirty-eight years. When Jesus saw him and knew he had been ill for a long time, he asked him, "Would you like to get well?"

John 5:3–6

Dear Lord,

I want to feel and look good again. I know I have not always taken care of my body and I am sorry. Please help me do better. I want to serve and please you, and I can do that best if I am well. Help me discover why my body is not functioning the way you intended. In Jesus's name, I pray. Amen.

	Breakfast	Lunch	Snack	Dinner
Food				
Time				
Three Hours Since Last Meal?				
Hungry?				
Feel an Emotion? Describe:				
Satisfied or Stuffed				
Digestive Issue?				
Poor Mental Clarity?				
Bad Mood?				

3

DAY 3: HEALTHY EATING GUIDELINES

The following healthy eating guidelines are my secret to maintaining optimal weight and brain health. This is a low-carbohydrate, low-glycemic, anti-inflammatory eating plan, which is the type of diet recommended for improving memory and cognition and preventing and reversing type 2 diabetes. You can obtain a printable version of these Healthy Eating Guidelines at SusanUNeal.com/appendix (appendix 5 of *7 Steps to Get Off of Sugar and Carbohydrates*).

Low-carbohydrate, anti-inflammatory dietary guidelines include:

- About 50 percent of food items are fresh organic vegetables.
- Eat one fresh, raw serving of low-glycemic fruit per day. Low-glycemic fruits include green apples, berries, cherries, pears, plums, and grapefruit.
- Do not always eat cooked foods. Eat a couple of servings of raw vegetables every day. Have a salad for lunch with either nuts or meat. When eating out, order a salad or coleslaw as sides, since both are raw.
- Another 25 percent of your daily food intake should come

from an animal or vegetable protein such as beans, nuts, and lean meats. Fish is exceptionally nutritious. Try to eat it once a week.

- A variety of different nuts and seeds are excellent sources of protein, minerals, and essential fatty acids.
- Avoid sugar, flour, rice, pasta, and bread. Instead, eat more fruits, vegetables, and low-glycemic grains such as quinoa and pearled barley.
- Beware of GMO Roundup Ready crops (most oat, corn, wheat, beet, and soy in the United States) that may contain residue from the carcinogen glyphosate (active ingredient in Roundup).[3] Therefore, buy only organic oat, corn, wheat, beet, and soy products.
- Do not eat sugary cereals. Instead, eat oatmeal, fruit, or granola. Be careful, as the sugar content of granola may be high. My favorite granola recipe appears in appendix 4 of *7 Steps to Get Off Sugar and Carbohydrates*.
- Try not to eat anything containing more than 10 grams of sugar in one serving.
- Eat nontraditional grains such as quinoa, amaranth, pearled barley, wild rice, and organic oats.
- Eat cultured foods such as kimchi, sauerkraut, and cultured plain Greek yogurt since they contain natural probiotics. Add one to two tablespoons of these foods to a meal twice a week or eat the yogurt as a snack. Personally I take a probiotic capsule every day.
- Replace sugary snacks with nuts, nut butter, dark chocolate, and plain Greek yogurt with berries.
- Replace condiments and sauces containing MSG or high-fructose corn syrup with spices, vinegar, and herbs.
- Replace fried foods with baked foods.

My additional healthy eating tips include:

- Make homemade granola from organic oats. For breakfast, I add fresh berries to a bowl of granola.
- Buy or whip up a flavorful dip like hummus or guacamole to eat with a platter of fresh vegetables (not chips or pita bread).
- Substitute beans for meat for some meals.
- Squeeze a slice of lemon and two drops of stevia into a glass of water. It is like drinking fresh lemonade.
- Boil eggs and keep them in the refrigerator for a snack.
- Chew your food thoroughly because this is where digestion begins.

Please try not to be overwhelmed by all of this information. Guide your eating with the 80/20 percent rule. *If you eat healthy 80 percent of the time and not so healthy 20 percent of the time, this will probably be an improvement.* I don't eat perfectly, but I try. With God's help, I try to follow these healthy eating guidelines a large percentage of the time.

	Breakfast	Lunch	Snack	Dinner
Food				
Time				
Three Hours Since Last Meal?				
Hungry?				
Feel an Emotion? Describe:				
Satisfied or Stuffed				
Digestive Issue?				
Poor Mental Clarity?				
Bad Mood?				

4

DAY 4: HOW DIFFERENT FOODS AFFECT YOUR BODY

Each of us has a unique body that reacts differently to various foods. High sugar content in foods causes problems in my system. Someone else may react negatively to the large gluten molecule of today's modern hybridized wheat. If you want to find out if you are gluten sensitive, either fast from gluten for a whole month, or take the Gluten Quiz at GlutenIntoleranceQuiz.com.

The purpose of this journal is to help you become aware of how different foods affect your body. Evaluate every item before you eat it to determine whether it is beneficial for you. Then pay attention to how you feel after you eat a specific food. By doing this, you can figure out what causes digestive problems, sleep disturbances, allergies, etc.

This is not a weight-loss program but a lifestyle change to improve your overall health so you feel better and therefore can serve God (and your family) to the best of your ability. If you evaluate everything you eat and ask yourself, "Did God create this food or did a food manufacturer make it to fatten their bottom line?" then you will begin changing your eating choices.

Many times we ignore what our body is trying to tell us. Instead, pay attention to it. Don't shrug off a symptom. Notice it and document it in the Issue Tracker at the beginning of this journal.

For decades my sister had to be close to a bathroom the day after she ate an unbeknownst type of food. It was terrible to be on a vacation and not know when this issue would occur. The problem was that she was sensitive to gluten and did not know it. She suffered for many years but, had she used a journal like this one, she could have figured out the offending food .

What type of undesirable symptom do you experience? Would you like to alleviate the symptom? (Fill out the Issue Tracker every time you experience the symptom.)

	Breakfast	Lunch	Snack	Dinner
Food				
Time				
Three Hours Since Last Meal?				
Hungry?				
Feel an Emotion? Describe:				
Satisfied or Stuffed				
Digestive Issue?				
Poor Mental Clarity?				
Bad Mood?				

5

DAY 5: MENU PLANNING

During this six-week period set aside time every week to plan your menu and grocery list. If you don't, you may end up eating unhealthy foods because you didn't take time to prepare properly. If you would like menus, recipes, and corresponding grocery lists, subscribe to my blog at SusanUNeal.com/healthy-living-blog.

While grocery shopping, shop along the edges of the store in the produce and refrigerated sections. Stay away from the center of the store where processed foods experience an extended shelf life. Remember, a long shelf life means the nutritional value of the food has been removed. If a food spoils, it is beneficial to the human body, but if it does not spoil, it contains no nutrients. Food in boxes and bags do not benefit the body but harm it.

What boxed or bagged food items do you need to eliminate?

_____

. . .

What obstacles do you face in creating a weekly menu and shopping list? How can you address these challenges to start a new way of food planning?

_____

_____

_____

Who in your family can you enlist to help you in menu planning and/or shopping? How can they partner with you to help?

_____

_____

_____

	Breakfast	Lunch	Snack	Dinner
Food				
Time				
Three Hours Since Last Meal?				
Hungry?				
Feel an Emotion? Describe:				
Satisfied or Stuffed				
Digestive Issue?				
Poor Mental Clarity?				
Bad Mood?				

DAY 6: JOURNAL TIME

	Breakfast	Lunch	Snack	Dinner
Food				
Time				
Three Hours Since Last Meal?				
Hungry?				
Feel an Emotion? Describe:				
Satisfied or Stuffed				
Digestive Issue?				
Poor Mental Clarity?				
Bad Mood?				

DAY 7: SABBATH REFLECTIONS

	Breakfast	Lunch	Snack	Dinner
Food				
Time				
Three Hours Since Last Meal?				
Hungry?				
Feel an Emotion? Describe:				
Satisfied or Stuffed				
Digestive Issue?				
Poor Mental Clarity?				
Bad Mood?				

PART II
WEEK 2

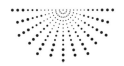

MENU PLAN

To ease the task of menu planning, I created a standard grocery list for the store I used. To create this list, initially I walked through the store and either wrote or dictated into my smartphone notes app the items I normally purchased on each grocery aisle. For example, I would start in the back of the store in the refrigerated section and would include eggs, butter, and coconut milk on the list for that aisle. Then I proceeded to the next aisle: cleaning supplies and paper products. I listed toilet paper, napkins, paper towels, paper plates, etc. And so on, until I compiled a master grocery.

At home, I typed out this list based on each grocery store aisle and the products I usually purchased. It took work to create this list, but it streamlined my grocery store planning for years.

Each week I printed a fresh new grocery list and my family knew that if we ran out of an item, they were supposed to circle it on the list or write it out. I made a rule to guide us—if it wasn't on the list, it didn't get purchased. I put the responsibility on them, not all on me.

Use the following chart to plan out your menu.

Meal	Monday	Tuesday
Breakfast		
Lunch		
Snack		
Dinner		

Meal	Wednesday	Thursday
Breakfast		
Lunch		
Snack		
Dinner		

Meal	Friday	Saturday
Breakfast		
Lunch		
Snack		
Dinner		

Meal	Sunday
Breakfast	
Lunch	
Snack	
Dinner	

WELL-BEING CHART

The following Well-Being Chart will help you determine how your habits affect your well-being. Record the number of hours you slept and add a Y for yes and N for no for the other items tracked below. Recognize if there is a correlation between your energy level and mood with the consumption of unhealthy foods. List those foods on the chart.

Your sleep and diet affect your brain. If you slept less than eight hours or ate unhealthy foods, color the box red in the Well-Being Chart. If you experience a day with high energy and clarity of mind color the corresponding boxes green.

Many of the symptoms listed in the Well-Being Chart (energy, brain fog, mood, anxiety, irritability, digestive issues) are affected by the foods you consume.

At the end of the week review your Daily Food Journals and compare it with your Well-Being Chart to determine how you did food wise along with the corresponding symptoms. When you color boxes red (negative symptoms) and green (positive symptoms) it is easier to figure out what type of food makes your body function well and vice-versa. When you find a food culprit, eliminate it from your diet.

Record the information below.

Days	8	9	10	11	12	13	14
Hours of Sleep							
Ate Unhealthy Foods: List the foods							
Binged							
Low Energy Level							
Brain Fog							
Bad Mood							
Anxiety							
Irritable							
Digestive Issues							
Physical Activity							
Probiotics							
Spent Time w/ God							

8

DAY 8: ACQUIRE KNOWLEDGE

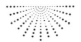

Have you ever found yourself eating something you thought was nutritious, only to find out later it wasn't? In our society it is difficult to navigate diet trends. In the 1980s, low-fat diets were the trend; now the ketogenic diet is popular. However, these eating methods seem to be the exact opposite. Which one is best?

Lack of knowledge is a key reason people fall into the trap of unintentionally eating the wrong types of food. When people gain knowledge, they recognize that their previous beliefs were false, and it becomes easier to overcome unhealthy eating habits. Acquiring knowledge regarding unhealthy versus healthy foods is crucial to making this lifestyle change. If you are serious about improving your health and weight, follow the seven simple steps in *7 Steps to Get Off Sugar and Carbohydrates* (see Day 11: Seven-Step Plan).

When you apply God's wisdom, along with accurate knowledge about today's food, you will improve your health and weight. Once you have the knowledge you need to make the right decision for your health, you'll be better equipped to take the next step, and the next, until you've changed your lifestyle. With your lifestyle change, you will live the abundant life Jesus wants you to experience, not a life filled with disease and unwanted, unhealthy symptoms.

. . .

My people are destroyed from lack of knowledge.

Hosea 4:6 (NIV)

	Breakfast	Lunch	Snack	Dinner
Food				
Time				
Three Hours Since Last Meal?				
Hungry?				
Feel an Emotion? Describe:				
Satisfied or Stuffed				
Digestive Issue?				
Poor Mental Clarity?				
Bad Mood?				

9

DAY 9: FOOD ADDICTION

The overabundance of delicacies in our society is hard to resist. Regrettably, people become addicted to sugar and carbs to the point that it causes excessive weight gain or health issues.

Sugar triggers the release of dopamine in the brain, which is part of our bodies' feel-good reward system. We enjoy the feeling of dopamine, so we keep eating carbs. At some point, an overconsumption of sugar and processed food rewires the brain's neural pathways and causes a person to become addicted.

The brain's hijacking triggers binge eating despite its consequences of weight gain and health problems. Therefore, getting off sugar is more complex than it may seem. It is no longer about willpower and self-discipline but a *biochemical addiction.*

Determining whether you are a food addict will help you understand yourself and enable you to effectively overcome this addiction. Take an online quiz to determine if you are addicted to food, by going to SusanUNeal.com/Resources. If your test was positive, I recommend you do the study in *Christian Study Guide for 7 Steps to Get Off Sugar and Carbohydrates.*

. . .

Do you eat in a manner you do not like? If yes, how?

_____

_____

_____

Do you think you have a food addiction? Journal your thoughts here:

_____

_____

_____

If you have a food addiction, what have the consequences been for you?

_____

_____

_____

. . .

Similarly, Paul struggled as indicated in this scripture:

The trouble is with me, for I am all too human, a slave to sin. I don't really understand myself, for I want to do what is right, but I don't do it. Instead, I do what I hate.

Romans 7:14–15

Dear Lord,

I know many of the foods I consume are not beneficial for me, but I can't seem to change. Please help me figure out what is going on inside of my body so I can gain control. It is nice to know that Paul struggled to do "what is right." Help me Lord to do what is right and pleasing in your sight. Jesus, through your holy name, I pray. Amen.

	Breakfast	Lunch	Snack	Dinner
Food				
Time				
Three Hours Since Last Meal?				
Hungry?				
Feel an Emotion? Describe:				
Satisfied or Stuffed				
Digestive Issue?				
Poor Mental Clarity?				
Bad Mood?				

DAY 10: CANDIDA

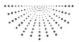

God made the human gastrointestinal (GI) system with the perfect balance of beneficial microorganisms. However, when a person consumes the standard American diet containing dyes, chemicals, excess sugar, and the residue of pesticides and herbicides, it disrupts the gut's equilibrium. The primary offender of this imbalance is antibiotics. They kill the good microbes and thereby, cause a bad guy — Candida—to overgrow. Candida makes a person crave sugar, alcohol, wheat, and processed foods because that is what it eats.

Candida Albicans, a type of yeast common in the gut, can grow roots into the lining of your GI system. The fungal overgrowth can create openings in the bowel walls, which is known as a leaky gut. These holes allow harmful microorganisms to enter the bloodstream. Our bodies don't recognize these particles, so our immune system creates antibodies, which cause food allergies and autoimmune diseases to develop.[4] An overgrowth of Candida also causes the abdomen to become distended.

When Candida spreads out of control, it acts like a parasite sucking the life and energy out of you. It is like a monster growing inside of you, craving sugar, and it is hard to fight its ever-increasing appetite. I had an overgrowth of Candida, so I know how hard it is to fight this culprit.

If you want to determine if you have a candida overgrowth in your gut, take the Candida Quiz at CandiQuiz.com. In addition, to you could take a simple spit test. First thing in the morning, before you drink anything or brush your teeth, spit into a glass of water. In one to three minutes, check the cup to see if any strings hang down from the spit—strings are a positive sign of Candida. The spit will resemble a jellyfish. If the water becomes cloudy or the saliva sinks to the bottom, this is also a sign of Candida. Healthy saliva floats on the top of the water with no strings hanging down.

To kill the bug in your gut (Candida) take an anti-Candida cleanse. Read the instructions on the cleanse package for how to administer it. Initially, I recommend taking the cleanse every other day for the first week to minimize lethargy and headaches. You will feel awful if the dead Candida is not quickly expelled from your colon. To avoid becoming constipated, drink plenty of water and increase the fiber in your diet.

The first three days you are on the cleanse, you may not feel well, but after a week you will begin to feel better than you have in a long time. You are just about to get the life back Jesus wants you to experience—one that is abundant and full.

If you would like more specific instructions about getting rid of Candida, get a copy of *7 Steps to Get Off Sugar and Carbohydrates* so you can start your journey to optimal health.

	Breakfast	Lunch	Snack	Dinner
Food				
Time				
Three Hours Since Last Meal?				
Hungry?				
Feel an Emotion? Describe:				
Satisfied or Stuffed				
Digestive Issue?				
Poor Mental Clarity?				
Bad Mood?				

DAY 11: SEVEN-STEP PLAN

Would you like to improve the way you feel and look while increasing your energy level and clarity of mind? How about losing weight naturally without going on a fad diet or buying prepared meals and supplements? You can achieve these results by implementing the following seven steps.

Seven Steps to Get Off Sugar and Carbs

Step 1. Decide to improve your health through proper nutrition.

Step 2. Acquire a support system and knowledge to help make a lifestyle change.

Step 3. Clean out your pantry and refrigerator by removing unhealthy foods and clean out your emotions with God.

Step 4. Purchase healthy foods and an anti-Candida cleanse.

Step 5. Plan for the date to begin changing your eating habits and implement the following seven-day eating plan listed below.

Step 6. Prepare and eat foods differently than you did before.

Step 7. Improve your health through continuing this new lifestyle never turning back to your old eating habits.

. . .

Seven-Day Eating Plan

Day 1: Drink your recommended amount of water per day. Stop eating sugar. Take a probiotic.

Day 2: Stop eating wheat.

Day 3: Do not eat processed foods out of boxes and bags. Eat 50 percent of your food fresh and raw. Follow the Healthy Eating Guidelines provided in appendix 5 of *7 Steps to Get Off Sugar and Carbohydrates*. Obtain a printable version of this plan at SusanUNeal.com/appendix.

Days 4 and 5: Focus on you. Rest, read, pray, and ask God to give you the willpower to succeed.

Day 6: Begin the anti-Candida cleanse.

Day 7: Get up and exercise.

These seven steps were taken from *7 Steps to Get Off Sugar and Carbohydrates*.

What steps do you plan to initiate?

	Breakfast	Lunch	Snack	Dinner
Food				
Time				
Three Hours Since Last Meal?				
Hungry?				
Feel an Emotion? Describe:				
Satisfied or Stuffed				
Digestive Issue?				
Poor Mental Clarity?				
Bad Mood?				

DAY 12: FOODS TO ELIMINATE

Understanding what foods are beneficial versus harmful is confusing today, especially since the food industry entices us through great marketing strategies and by adding addictive ingredients. It is far better to eat foods as close to their value at harvest—the way God made them—rather than processed foods.

You should eliminate the following foods from your diet:

- wheat—hybridized and most humans can't digest the gluten
- white flour—stripped of its nutrients
- sugar—addictive and raises blood-sugar levels and predisposes a person to diabetes
- corn syrup, also called high-fructose corn syrup— inexpensive alternative to sugar with the same devastating effects
- white rice—stripped of its nutrients
- corn (except organic)—most are GMO Roundup Ready crops and may contain the carcinogen glyphosate
- milk products—denatured of its nutritional value to extend

its shelf life and since it doesn't contain its natural enzymes human beings cannot properly digest it

- artificial sweeteners—causes a person to crave sweets
- processed meats—the World Health Organization classified processed meats (hot dogs, ham, bacon, sausage, and some deli meats) as a group 1 carcinogen[5]
- vegetable oils except for coconut and olive oil—most vegetable oils contain omega 6 fatty acids, which promote inflammation in the human body
- processed foods contained in boxes and bags—the nutrients and fiber are removed to increase their shelf life
- canned goods—lined with Bisphenol (BPA), which is a hormone disruptor, prevent erosion of the can
- margarine—contains trans-fat, which increases the risk of heart disease, and free radicals, which contribute to numerous health problems including cancer
- sugar-sweetened drinks, fruit juices—addictive, raise blood-sugar levels, and predispose a person to diabetes

By reducing or eliminating these foods you will improve the health of your body. For a complete explanation as to why you should stop eating these foods, read Step 3: Clean Out the Pantry and Refrigerator of *7 Steps to Get Off Sugar and Carbohydrates*.

	Breakfast	Lunch	Snack	Dinner
Food				
Time				
Three Hours Since Last Meal?				
Hungry?				
Feel an Emotion? Describe:				
Satisfied or Stuffed				
Digestive Issue?				
Poor Mental Clarity?				
Bad Mood?				

13

DAY 13: JOURNAL TIME

	Breakfast	Lunch	Snack	Dinner
Food				
Time				
Three Hours Since Last Meal?				
Hungry?				
Feel an Emotion? Describe:				
Satisfied or Stuffed				
Digestive Issue?				
Poor Mental Clarity?				
Bad Mood?				

14

DAY 14: SABBATH REFLECTIONS

	Breakfast	Lunch	Snack	Dinner
Food				
Time				
Three Hours Since Last Meal?				
Hungry?				
Feel an Emotion? Describe:				
Satisfied or Stuffed				
Digestive Issue?				
Poor Mental Clarity?				
Bad Mood?				

PART III
WEEK 3

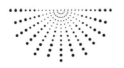

MENU PLAN

WEEKLY MENU PLANNING

This is an example of my cooking plan for a week. I cooked on Sunday and Monday and had leftovers (from Sunday) to be served on Tuesday. Wednesday we all ate at church, and Thursday I served leftovers from Monday. To liven up a leftover, I would cook one new item (such as a vegetable) to be served with the previous meal, and this new item gave the meal new interest. Two nights of cooking took care of four meals.

Every week I made a large, fresh, raw salad (broccoli salad, beet salad, cole slaw, salad with lettuce) and I ate that for my lunch throughout the week. I have over fifty recipes in the printable version of appendix 4 from *7 Steps to Get Off Sugar and Carbohydrates* at Susan-UNeal.com/appendix. For my children's lunch boxes, I tried to include one fresh fruit and vegetable each day.

Use the following chart to plan out your weekly menu.

Meal	Monday	Tuesday
Breakfast		
Lunch		
Snack		
Dinner		

Meal	Wednesday	Thursday
Breakfast		
Lunch		
Snack		
Dinner		

Meal	Friday	Saturday
Breakfast		
Lunch		
Snack		
Dinner		

Meal	Sunday
Breakfast	
Lunch	
Snack	
Dinner	

WELL-BEING CHART

The following Well-Being Chart will help you determine how your habits affect your well-being. Record the number of hours you slept and add a Y for yes and N for no for the other items tracked below. Recognize if there is a correlation between your energy level and mood with the consumption of unhealthy foods. List those foods on the chart.

Your sleep and diet affect your brain. If you slept less than eight hours or ate unhealthy foods, color the box red in the Well-Being Chart. If you experience a day with high energy and clarity of mind color the corresponding boxes green.

Many of the symptoms listed in the Well-Being Chart (energy, brain fog, mood, anxiety, irritability, digestive issues) are affected by the foods you consume.

At the end of the week review your Daily Food Journals and compare it with your Well-Being Chart to determine how you did food wise along with the corresponding symptoms. When you color boxes red (negative symptoms) and green (positive symptoms) it is easier to figure out what type of food makes your body function well and vice-versa. When you find a food culprit, eliminate it from your diet.

Please complete the information below.

Days	15	16	17	18	19	20	21
Hours of Sleep							
Ate Unhealthy Foods: List the foods							
Binged							
Low Energy Level							
Brain Fog							
Bad Mood							
Anxiety							
Irritable							
Digestive Issues							
Physical Activity							
Probiotics							
Spent Time w/ God							

15

DAY 15: ACCOUNTABILITY/PRAYER PARTNER

Acquiring a support system is integral to attaining success as you change your lifestyle. Therefore, ask someone to be your accountability and prayer partner. But first pray and ask God to give you wisdom to choose the right person.

That person should be someone who can understand the struggles you face but will not merely give you platitudes or think you should be able to "just do it." Your accountability partner should be one who will not give you permission to keep up your bad habits but will be both empathetic and truthful with you. Also, make sure this person is a Christian, so they can give you biblical advice and feel comfortable praying with you.

When someone understands how you feel, you are validated in your struggles, so it is helpful to reach out to a friend during this journey. Having a friend for accountability whom you can call when temptation arises is key to your success. It is powerful when someone speaks the truth in love.

Pray with your friend. The security of knowing this person prays for you is comforting. The following scripture confirms we should share trials and confess our sins to one another.

. . .

Confess your sins to each other and pray for each other so that you may be healed.

James 5:16

Dear heavenly Father,

Please help me to find the perfect prayer and accountability partner—one whom I can open up to and share my thoughts, struggles, and feelings. Thank you, Lord. Through Jesus's name I pray. Amen.

Who are you going to ask to be your accountability/prayer partner? When do you plan to ask this person?

What other type of support would be beneficial?

	Breakfast	Lunch	Snack	Dinner
Food				
Time				
Three Hours Since Last Meal?				
Hungry?				
Feel an Emotion? Describe:				
Satisfied or Stuffed				
Digestive Issue?				
Poor Mental Clarity?				
Bad Mood?				

16

DAY 16: TEMPTATION AND THE SWORD OF THE SPIRIT

When it comes to food, each of us struggles with temptation. I tend to overindulge with popcorn. While watching a movie, slowly but surely the whole tub disappears. So it is better for me to purchase a smaller portion. That's how I handle my temptation. You also need to figure out how to handle your food temptation.

What food struggle did you experience recently and how did you handle it? What would you do differently?

. . .

What time of day do you experience the most temptation?

Where were you when you were most tempted?

Was anyone with you when you were tempted?

Did you experience a strong emotion before you ate an unhealthy food? If yes, what was the feeling? Have you experienced this before?

. . .

As you figure out how to fight food temptation, record your strategies in Appendix 2: My Battle Strategies Plan. Then refer back to them as needed.

Sword of the Spirit

One of the ways to fight food addiction is through scripture. Appendix 1 of *7 Steps to Get Off Sugar and Carbohydrates* includes Bible verses to recite to tap into God's power and strength. You can obtain a printable version of this appendix at SusanUNeal.com/appendix. If you are addicted to sugar and carbohydrates, you need God's superpower.

Find a specific Bible verse to oppose your food issue and write it on an index card. Keep it with you until you memorize it. Speak the verse out loud every time you feel the urge to eat unhealthy foods.

When you choose to learn God's Word it will affect you positively in ways you can't imagine. We are supposed to store his word in our hearts. If we do we can draw upon them when the enemy whispers lies. Store the sword of the Spirit in your mind, so you can defeat Satan, and successfully achieve your goals.

I have hidden your word in my heart
    that I might not sin against you.

Psalm 119:11

Choose your strategic Bible verse and write it here. It is your sword; carry it with you and unsheathe it as needed.

. . .

	Breakfast	Lunch	Snack	Dinner
Food				
Time				
Three Hours Since Last Meal?				
Hungry?				
Feel an Emotion? Describe:				
Satisfied or Stuffed				
Digestive Issue?				
Poor Mental Clarity?				
Bad Mood?				

17

DAY 17: PRAYER

Prayer is an essential component of the arsenal God gave us, as Paul indicated in Ephesians 6:18, "And pray in the Spirit on all occasions with all kinds of prayers and requests" (NIV). To make the lifestyle changes necessary to improve your health, access your heavenly father through prayer. Prayer breaks down the resistance you may experience as you make these changes.

When Jesus was in Gethsemane, he prayed to his Father. We need to follow Jesus's example. God wants to communicate with us, and through prayer we receive his power to face our struggles. Ask God to give you a willing spirit to surrender to him, and replace your desire for food with the desire to please and serve him.

Jesus's brother told us:

The earnest prayer of a righteous man has great power and wonderful results.

James 5:16 (TLB)

Spend a few minutes telling God how you feel and what you desire. Ask him to help you achieve your goals. Tell him about your disappointments, and ask him to empower you during your struggles.

_____

_____

_____

_____

_____

_____

_____

_____

_____

	Breakfast	Lunch	Snack	Dinner
Food				
Time				
Three Hours Since Last Meal?				
Hungry?				
Feel an Emotion? Describe:				
Satisfied or Stuffed				
Digestive Issue?				
Poor Mental Clarity?				
Bad Mood?				

18

DAY 18: MEDITATING WITH GOD

Most mornings I sit in the living room with my cup of tea and spend time with God. I close my eyes and focus on the Lord. While I draw in a deep breath, my mind drifts. Situations I didn't realize were significant to me become apparent. Emotions I suppressed resurface. The Lord purges and percolates my whole being to reveal what's truly important. Spending a few minutes every morning with him brings peace to my mind and soul.

Christian meditation is beneficial to our overall well-being. Mindfulness exercises such as Christian yoga train a person's mind to pay attention to cravings without reacting to them. When a person becomes more mindful, she notices why she wants to indulge but can move through the feeling without reacting to it. I created several Christian yoga products including DVDs, books, and card decks, available at ChristianYoga.com, which could help you become more mindful.

I will meditate about your glory, splendor, majesty, and miracles.

Psalm 145:5 (TLB)

Meditate on the Lord and journal your thoughts.

_____

_____

_____

_____

_____

_____

_____

_____

	Breakfast	Lunch	Snack	Dinner
Food				
Time				
Three Hours Since Last Meal?				
Hungry?				
Feel an Emotion? Describe:				
Satisfied or Stuffed				
Digestive Issue?				
Poor Mental Clarity?				
Bad Mood?				

DAY 19: FIVE-STEPS TO FREEDOM FROM ADDICTION

If you are addicted to food, you can gain freedom by implementing the five steps in the plan below. You can obtain a printable version of this plan from appendix 8 in *7 Steps to Get Off Sugar and Carbohydrates* by going to SusanUNeal.com/appendix. Post the five-step plan on your refrigerator or bathroom mirror and use it when tempted to overeat unhealthy foods.

1. Name what controls you.

Name the thing controlling you—food addiction, anxiety, eating disorder, depression, etc.—whatever it may be, and declare (out loud) Jesus Christ is your Lord in its place![6]

Stand up to the evil spirit who brought bondage into your life by saying, "Evil spirit, you won't lord over me or entice me through (insert your addiction) anymore. Jesus is my Lord!" A person obtains spiritual power and authority through Christ. Declare that the spiritual powers of darkness will not have lordship over your life. They will not rule you, govern your behavior, capture your thought life, or lead you into temptation and sin because "the one who is in you is greater than the one who is in the world" (1 John 4:4 NIV).

. . .

2. Submit yourself completely to God.

"Submit yourself, then, to God. Resist the devil, and he will flee from you." James 4:7 (NIV)

There is a secret to resisting the devil—you must first submit yourself to God. How in the world do you do that? In my experience, you no longer do your will but God's will by submitting your life to him.

3. Use the name of Jesus.

In the book of Acts, the apostles healed and worked miracles in the name of Jesus. Use Jesus's name as Peter did in Acts 3:6: "In the name of Jesus Christ of Nazareth, *walk!*" (TLB). Using the name of Jesus is key to binding the spiritual nature of an addiction, because then you operate under Jesus's authority.

4. Use the Word of God.

The Holy Spirit inside of you is stronger than Satan and his demons. By using the name of Jesus, you are not only under his authority but you can speak with his authority. You are much better armed than Satan. Now is the time to stand up to him, strip him of his weapons, and kick him out of your life through the Word of God! Speak out loud, "In the name of Jesus, you won't oppress me anymore. I bind your power in the name of Jesus and by the Word of God."

5. Praise God and practice gratitude.

When you praise God and thank him for his blessings, the demonic forces won't hang around. Fill your mind, heart, and body with the Spirit of God by putting the right things in your spirit. Listen to praise music; read the Bible and pray; memorize scripture; attend church, Sunday school, or a Bible study. Also start doing more to help others. Performing acts of service and helping others fills your heart with honorable feelings and humility. Every day write in your journal about all you can praise God for and thank him.

Beat the addiction by declaring Bible verses out loud. Stomp the spiritual nature of the addiction into the ground by singing praises to God. The devil can't stand to be around someone who worships the Lord. Become God's warrior by using his mighty unseen weapons. Paul advises:

It is true that I am an ordinary, weak human being, but I don't use human plans and methods to win my battles. I use God's mighty weapons, not those made by men, to knock down the devil's strongholds.

2 Corinthians 10:3–4 (TLB)

You are God's mighty conqueror!

How do you intend to put this plan into action?

	Breakfast	Lunch	Snack	Dinner
Food				
Time				
Three Hours Since Last Meal?				
Hungry?				
Feel an Emotion? Describe:				
Satisfied or Stuffed				
Digestive Issue?				
Poor Mental Clarity?				
Bad Mood?				

20

DAY 20: JOURNAL TIME

	Breakfast	Lunch	Snack	Dinner
Food				
Time				
Three Hours Since Last Meal?				
Hungry?				
Feel an Emotion? Describe:				
Satisfied or Stuffed				
Digestive Issue?				
Poor Mental Clarity?				
Bad Mood?				

21

DAY 21: SABBATH REFLECTIONS

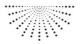

	Breakfast	Lunch	Snack	Dinner
Food				
Time				
Three Hours Since Last Meal?				
Hungry?				
Feel an Emotion? Describe:				
Satisfied or Stuffed				
Digestive Issue?				
Poor Mental Clarity?				
Bad Mood?				

PART IV
WEEK 4

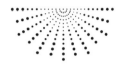

MENU PLAN

WEEKLY MENU PLANNING

Think of foods as being dead or alive. Food from a bag sitting on the shelf for months is dead and does not give your body any of the nutrients it needs to be healthy. A fresh piece of fruit contains essential vitamins, minerals, and fiber that the human body needs.

The fiber in fruits and vegetables you consume fills your stomach and tells your body you are full. When the fiber is removed, as in processed foods, it takes a larger quantity of food to become full. Also, the fiber in fruit slows digestion, which reduces the effects of sugar in raising your blood-sugar levels. As you eliminate processed foods from you diet you should consume more whole, organic fruits, vegetables, whole grains (oats, brown rice, quinoa, barley), beans, fish, and meat. Your body will thank you for nourishing it properly and will respond by healing itself.

Today, I look at any food and assess whether or not it is good for me. If a person primarily eats dead food, how does the body get the proper nutrients it needs? How can your body replace old cells with healthy new ones if you don't give it the essential vitamins and minerals it requires? If the body does not receive proper nutrition to perform the functions required for life and regeneration, it will break down. If cells within the human body replicate incorrectly cancer will develop.

Use the following chart to plan out your weekly menu.

Meal	Monday	Tuesday
Breakfast		
Lunch		
Snack		
Dinner		

Meal	Wednesday	Thursday
Breakfast		
Lunch		
Snack		
Dinner		

Meal	Friday	Saturday
Breakfast		
Lunch		
Snack		
Dinner		

Meal	Sunday
Breakfast	
Lunch	
Snack	
Dinner	

WELL-BEING CHART

The following Well-Being Chart will help you determine how habits affect your well-being. Record the number of hours you slept and add a Y for yes and N for no for the other items tracked below. Recognize if there is a correlation between your energy level and mood with the consumption of unhealthy foods. List those foods on the chart.

Your sleep and diet affect your brain. If you slept less than eight hours or ate unhealthy foods, color the box red in the Well-Being Chart. If you experience a day with high energy and clarity of mind color the corresponding boxes green.

Many of the symptoms listed in the Well-Being Chart (energy, brain fog, mood, anxiety, irritability, digestive issues) are affected by the foods you consume.

At the end of the week review your Daily Food Journals and compare it with your Well-Being Chart to determine how you did food wise along with the corresponding symptoms. When you color boxes red (negative symptoms) and green (positive symptoms) it is easier to figure out what type of food makes your body function well and vice-versa. When you find a food culprit, eliminate it from your diet.

Please complete the information below.

Days	22	23	24	25	26	27	28
Hours of Sleep							
Ate Unhealthy Foods: List the foods							
Binged							
Low Energy Level							
Brain Fog							
Bad Mood							
Anxiety							
Irritable							
Digestive Issues							
Physical Activity							
Probiotics							
Spent Time w/ God							

22

DAY 22: EMOTIONAL ISSUES WITH FOOD

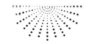

For most of us, food and emotions are intrinsically tied together, so we need to do an emotional assessment and identify whether food brings us comfort.

If you need additional support figuring out emotional eating and how to resolve it, purchase my course, 7 Steps to Reclaim Your Health and Optimal Weight (https://susanuneal.com/courses/7-steps-to-get-off-sugar-and-carbs-course). In this course I walk you through the steps to change your eating habits once and for all.

How do you look at food? Are you using food to comfort yourself or meet an emotional need, or do you think of food as a necessity to keep your body functioning?

_____

_____

Do you turn to food to help you deal with life's challenges?

. . .

_____

God gave us food to nourish our bodies. Yet food can be used for the wrong reasons. We may eat because we are sad, bored, stressed out, depressed, or happy. As we engage in emotional eating, we turn to food, instead of God, to appease ourselves. If we feel abandoned, food can be our friend. We can swallow our angry feelings with food, instead of feeling the emotions we don't want to deal with. Food can provide an emotional escape from negative feelings.

Do you use food to escape from emotional issues? If yes, how?

_____

_____

_____

In your Daily Food Journal chart there is a column to document if you ate because you were hungry and if three hours passed since your last meal. On average it takes two to three hours for your previous meal to digest unless you ate fruit only. Each day determine if you are eating because of hunger or for some other reason. If you are not hungry, document why you are eating.

Do you have a deep emotional wound that needs healing? If you do, journal and talk to God about it. Is there someone you need to forgive? Maybe you have a big hole in your heart that you are filling with food.

God is our ultimate healer, take your wounds to him and ask him to heal you.

_____

_____

_____

If you have an emotional connection with food, please consider using the *Christian Study Guide for 7 Steps to Get Off Sugar and Carbohydrates.* Whether you do this study by yourself or with a group, it will help you go more in-depth to resolve emotional issues once and for all. Please join my closed Facebook group, 7 Steps to Get Off Sugar, Carbs, and Gluten and share with me how you are doing. If you would like healthy living tips please like my Facebook page at Face-book.com/HealthyLivingSeries/.

Your weight does not determine your value to God. Your body is the temple of the Holy Spirit. Call on the Holy Spirit to empower you to change. With God's help, you can overcome and succeed.

The eyes of the LORD search the whole earth in order to strengthen those whose hearts are fully committed to him.

2 Chronicles 16:9

Dear Lord,

Please help me to understand my emotional connection with food. I want to replace my appetite with a desire for you. Please fill me with your Spirit and strengthen me. Turning to you first is what I want to do. Jesus, through your name, I pray. Amen.

	Breakfast	Lunch	Snack	Dinner
Food				
Time				
Three Hours Since Last Meal?				
Hungry?				
Feel an Emotion? Describe:				
Satisfied or Stuffed				
Digestive Issue?				
Poor Mental Clarity?				
Bad Mood?				

23

DAY 23: CLEAN OUT YOUR EMOTIONS

In this journal, record your thoughts as they relate to your consumption of food. The last two days of every week's devotions provide blank pages for you to write on. Figure out what triggers you to eat (when you are not hungry) and journal when you eat because of a negative emotion. This may help you identify dysfunctional eating behaviors.

What food problems have been with you since childhood? Take some time with God and record what instances from your past resulted in the way you eat today.

_____

_____

_____

. . .

After you pinpoint your food issue, bring it to God and be honest with him about what you experience. Each time you recognize that you engage in emotional eating, clean out your emotions with the Lord so you can disengage the connection between eating and feelings.

Begin the process of cleaning out your emotions by telling God what you think is the origin of your unhealthy eating habit and ask him to help you heal from any emotional scars.

Changing your eating habits is not an overnight process. The more extended the period of unhealthy eating, the longer it will take to reset your body and mind. But step-by-step you can reprogram your body, mind, and spirit. Creating a support system and journaling are vital components to your success. You are on the path to recover your health and weight!

	Breakfast	Lunch	Snack	Dinner
Food				
Time				
Three Hours Since Last Meal?				
Hungry?				
Feel an Emotion? Describe:				
Satisfied or Stuffed				
Digestive Issue?				
Poor Mental Clarity?				
Bad Mood?				

24

DAY 24: BOREDOM/STRESS EATING

Sometimes we engage in mindless eating, where we munch on something without being hungry (for me it's popcorn). When a person is bored, she may look in the refrigerator or pantry but can't find anything appealing. If this happens to you, food is not what you need. First, drink two glasses of water, as you may be thirsty and don't realize it. Next, your soul may be longing for a connection with God, so spend time with him.

Journal your thoughts here.

_____ _____

_____

_____ _____

. . .

Stress also causes a person to turn to food. Determine the stressors (things that cause you stress) in your life. Can you do something about the stressors? Pray to God and ask him to enlighten you. Ask your accountability partner or support group for help and prayer in dealing with your stressors.

How do you cope with stress? Do you tend to deal with it through undesirable eating habits? If so, recognize this and choose to do something about your stress level. Some stress-relieving activities include getting a massage, journaling, calling a friend, and watching a movie.

Don't worry about anything; instead, pray about everything. Tell God what you need, and thank him for all he has done. Then you will experience God's peace, which exceeds anything we can understand. His peace will guard your hearts and minds as you live in Christ Jesus.

Philippians 4:6–7

I created an equation to correspond with this verse: Don't worry + Pray + Thank God + Abide in Jesus = God's Peace. Ask God to help you not worry, pray, thank him, and abide in Jesus so you can experience his peace that transcends all understanding.

Lord,

I need your help to stop worrying. Help me to turn to you and pray instead of turning to worldly things like food. I want to remember to thank you for even the small things. But most of all give me faith to believe Jesus is with me and I can call on him at any time to give me strength to overcome my battle with food. Thank you in advance for answering my prayer. Through Jesus's holy and precious name, I pray. Amen.

	Breakfast	Lunch	Snack	Dinner
Food				
Time				
Three Hours Since Last Meal?				
Hungry?				
Feel an Emotion? Describe:				
Satisfied or Stuffed				
Digestive Issue?				
Poor Mental Clarity?				
Bad Mood?				

DAY 25: BINGING

Overeating is unhealthy, and when that becomes a habit, eventually a person becomes addicted to food and can't stop eating it. In turn, this causes binging. Binge eating occurs when you can't stop eating an item even though you want to. You can't control yourself. Afterward, you regret what you did. If you binge, be sure to journal afterward in the Binge Eating Tracker. Determine your feelings before you binged and what temptation led you down that path.

Figure out your trigger and record it in the Temptation/Struggle Log. When you understand what tempts you, you can learn to avoid it.

What did you tell yourself that validated why it was okay to overeat?

_____

_____

. . .

Ask God to help you not to overindulge to the point of gluttony.

_____

_____

After binging, ask God to forgive you and help you not to binge again. Record your experience in the blank pages of the sixth or seventh day of each week's journal. Once you ask for forgiveness, God chooses not to remember your sins, as indicated in Hebrews 8:12: "And I will be merciful to them in their wrongdoings, and I will remember their sins no more" (TLB). Don't fret over a stumble. Get up and try again using the Five Spiritual Steps to Freedom from Addiction (day 19). You can get a printable copy of this plan at SusanUNeal.com/appendix; it is also in appendix 8 from *7 Steps to Get Off Sugar and Carbohydrates*.

If you record every incident of overeating in the Binge Eating Tracker and implement the five-step plan every time you binge, you will overcome and experience success. Retraining your mind is like disciplining a child; consistency is vital to transformation.

Don't copy the behavior and customs of this world, but let God transform you into a new person by changing the way you think. Then you will learn to know God's will for you, which is good and pleasing and perfect.

Romans 12:2

Father, Please transform me by changing the way I think. I need your power to beat this addiction to food. I can't do this without your transforming power, so I surrender my addiction to you. I believe you will instill your strength in me to meet this challenge so I can overcome it. I will replace my desire for food with your "pleasing and perfect" plan for me. Please remind me to seek you first and not food. Through Jesus's name I pray. Amen.

	Breakfast	Lunch	Snack	Dinner
Food				
Time				
Three Hours Since Last Meal?				
Hungry?				
Feel an Emotion? Describe:				
Satisfied or Stuffed				
Digestive Issue?				
Poor Mental Clarity?				
Bad Mood?				

26

DAY 26: FIGHT FOOD TEMPTATION

Every morning, first spend time with God. Then plan your day by determining your menu and what food struggles you might encounter. Decide how you will fight food temptation. Select a scripture verse to help you resist, and begin the day by reciting it out loud.

When you recognize temptation, remove yourself from the area containing the food, and record the enticement in the Temptation/Struggle Log at the beginning of this journal. Some strategies for resisting temptation include:

- pray
- go for a walk
- recite your Bible verse
- call your prayer partner
- drink two glasses of water
- listen to praise music and worship God
- spend time with and meditate about God

Record other helpful strategies you develop in Appendix 2: My Battle Strategies Plan. For a list of Food Addiction Battle Strategies, see appendix 1. Also, when you are tempted, think about how far you have come in overcoming your food addiction and whether you want to experience the withdrawal symptoms again.

Write down five reasons why you do not want to eat unhealthy food.

_____

_____

_____

_____

_____

"And call on me in the day of trouble;
   I will deliver you, and you will honor me."

Psalm 50:15 (NIV)

Dear Lord,

Help me to plan my day, spend time with you, and successfully fight any food temptation I may encounter today. Jesus, give me strength. In your name I pray. Amen.

	Breakfast	Lunch	Snack	Dinner
Food				
Time				
Three Hours Since Last Meal?				
Hungry?				
Feel an Emotion? Describe:				
Satisfied or Stuffed				
Digestive Issue?				
Poor Mental Clarity?				
Bad Mood?				

DAY 27: JOURNAL TIME

	Breakfast	Lunch	Snack	Dinner
Food				
Time				
Three Hours Since Last Meal?				
Hungry?				
Feel an Emotion? Describe:				
Satisfied or Stuffed				
Digestive Issue?				
Poor Mental Clarity?				
Bad Mood?				

DAY 28: SABBATH REFLECTIONS

	Breakfast	Lunch	Snack	Dinner
Food				
Time				
Three Hours Since Last Meal?				
Hungry?				
Feel an Emotion? Describe:				
Satisfied or Stuffed				
Digestive Issue?				
Poor Mental Clarity?				
Bad Mood?				

PART V
WEEK 5

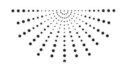

MENU PLAN

WEEKLY MENU PLANNING

Meals don't have to be complex. It wasn't complicated for Adam and Eve in the garden of Eden. They picked a piece of fruit or a vegetable and ate it. It doesn't have to be difficult for us either. Instead of making an elaborate meal, eat fresh, raw vegetables, which cost less and are better for you than processed, sugar-laden products.

Farmer's markets are great venues to find fresh, local produce. It is best to eat locally grown fruit and vegetables. Buy a potato and bake it with the following toppings: olive oil, broccoli, scallions, and sea salt with kelp (seaweed). The baked potato is better for you than a bag of potato chips. Eat foods closer to the form they were in when they came out of the garden.

Check labels and try not to eat foods with more than five ingredients and 10 grams of sugar per serving. The American Heart Association recommends you limit your calories from sugar to no more than half of your total calories, which is a lot. For most women in the US that should be no more than 24 grams of sugar or 100 calories per day. For men it is 36 grams of sugar or 150 calories from sugar per day.

If you can't pronounce an ingredient, your body probably won't recognize it as food either. Begin to simplify the foods you consume.

For example, eat two hard-boiled eggs for breakfast, a whole avocado for lunch, and an apple for a snack. Ask yourself, "Did the food I am about to eat exist in the garden of Eden?" Food doesn't have to be complicated.

Meal	Monday	Tuesday
Breakfast		
Lunch		
Snack		
Dinner		

Meal	Wednesday	Thursday
Breakfast		
Lunch		
Snack		
Dinner		

Meal	Friday	Saturday
Breakfast		
Lunch		
Snack		
Dinner		

Meal	Sunday
Breakfast	
Lunch	
Snack	
Dinner	

WELL-BEING CHART

The following Well-Being Chart will help you determine how habits affect your well-being. Record the number of hours you slept and add a Y for yes and N for no for the other items tracked below. Recognize if there is a correlation between your energy level and mood with the consumption of unhealthy foods. List those foods on the chart.

Your sleep and diet affect your brain. If you slept less than eight hours or ate unhealthy foods, color the box red in the Well-Being Chart. If you experience a day with high energy and clarity of mind color the corresponding boxes green.

Many of the symptoms listed in the Well-Being Chart (energy, brain fog, mood, anxiety, irritability, digestive issues) are affected by the foods you consume.

At the end of the week review your Daily Food Journals and compare it with your Well-Being Chart to determine how you did food wise along with the corresponding symptoms. When you color boxes red (negative symptoms) and green (positive symptoms) it is easier to figure out what type of food makes your body function well and vice-versa. When you find a food culprit, eliminate it from your diet.

Please complete the information below.

Days	29	30	31	32	33	34	35
Hours of Sleep							
Ate Unhealthy Foods: List the foods							
Binged							
Low Energy Level							
Brain Fog							
Bad Mood							
Anxiety							
Irritable							
Digestive Issues							
Physical Activity							
Probiotics							
Spent Time w/ God							

29

DAY 29: DIGESTIVE ISSUES

It is essential to notice how your body reacts to different foods. If you experience digestive problems, keep track of what you ate before the symptom—in the Issue Tracker at the beginning of this journal. Notice if you consistently belch after a particular type of food. If you do you may need to avoid this food or take a digestive enzyme (from a health food store). As we age or damage our GI tract, a person may not secrete enough digestive enzymes to break down their food properly. However, you can take an enzyme when you eat food so it will be digested properly.

Note whether you have problems digesting wheat or dairy, as these two products are the usual offenders. My culprit was sunflower and sesame seeds. I normally added those seeds to my homemade granola, but I often belched after I ate the granola. When I documented what I ate, I figured out what caused the digestive issue. When I eliminated those seeds from the recipe, my indigestion ceased.

Today's wheat is hybridized to the point that the gluten molecule is so large most humans cannot digest it. Therefore it is a major digestive offender. If you need to take an antacid, I recommend you stop eating wheat and see if your symptoms disappear.

. . .

What type of digestive issues do you experience?

_____

	Breakfast	Lunch	Snack	Dinner
Food				
Time				
Three Hours Since Last Meal?				
Hungry?				
Feel an Emotion? Describe:				
Satisfied or Stuffed				
Digestive Issue?				
Poor Mental Clarity?				
Bad Mood?				

30

DAY 30: FOODS THAT CAUSE INFLAMMATION

Some medical literature claims inflammation is the root of chronic disease. Where do you think inflammation comes from? It generates from what we put into our bodies and most likely from food.

We eat many foods that are far from the products they were when first harvested. The human body does not recognize some of these so-called foods and so it reacts negatively and causes inflammation. Inflammation causes a wide-range of adverse effects across many systems in the body. It is critical to identify what food is causing a negative reaction in your body.

This journal will help you figure out this part of the puzzle. When you experience a negative physical symptom, record it in the Issue Tracker. Also note what foods you ate within the past twelve hours. You may recognize a pattern regarding a specific type of food. For me it was dairy; this food always caused me to experience congestion and postnasal drip at night.

If you think a specific food may be causing problematic symptoms in your body, eliminate it for at least a week. When you reintroduce it, be sure to record in your journal what symptoms you experience. If you would like me to coach you during this process, I am a Health and

Wellness Coach and I offer services at SusanUNeal.com/Health-Coaching.

What foods do you think may be causing you a problem?

_____

	Breakfast	Lunch	Snack	Dinner
Food				
Time				
Three Hours Since Last Meal?				
Hungry?				
Feel an Emotion? Describe:				
Satisfied or Stuffed				
Digestive Issue?				
Poor Mental Clarity?				
Bad Mood?				

DAY 31: FOOD SUBSTITUTES

As you begin to improve your eating habits, you need to find food substitutes. Many unhealthy food choices can be replaced with healthy alternatives that are whole, unprocessed, and natural. Here is a list of suggestions.

Sugar Substitutes

In the following list the best natural sugar substitutes are ranked based on their glycemic index:

stevia-0

monk fruit sweetener-0

xylitol-12

agave-15

coconut sugar-35

honey-50

maple syrup-54

Choose a natural, low-glycemic sweetener that you can live with and use it sparingly.

. . .

Pasta Substitutes

Cook spaghetti squash, shirataki, quinoa or chickpea noodles, or spiralize zucchini.

Milk Substitutes

It is best not to consume milk products. However, several healthy dairy substitutes include almond, cashew, coconut, and pea milk. I enjoy the flavor of toasted coconut almond blend, which combines both of these kinds of milk.

Which sugar, milk, or pasta substitute listed above will you commit to try?

_____

What type of foods have you eliminated so far? What food do you want to eliminate?

_____

Pray and ask God to give you the motivation and strength to make a positive lifestyle changes.

_____

. . .

	Breakfast	Lunch	Snack	Dinner
Food				
Time				
Three Hours Since Last Meal?				
Hungry?				
Feel an Emotion? Describe:				
Satisfied or Stuffed				
Digestive Issue?				
Poor Mental Clarity?				
Bad Mood?				

DAY 32: TIPS FOR A HEALTHIER LIFESTYLE

Simple changes like drinking plenty of water or eating only until you are full will help you transition into this new way of eating. Suggestions for choosing healthy foods when eating out are always needed. The following tips should assist you to successfully make healthy lifestyle changes.

Only Eat Until You're Full

As you prepare to eat healthier, one positive change you can make is to pay attention to the sensation of fullness as you eat. Some individuals may not be in touch with that feeling anymore. Focus on recognizing when you are full so you do not overeat. You may have to change some of your mealtime habits as well. Eat slowly, chew your food thoroughly, and pay attention to how the food tastes.

When you eat processed foods, versus meals you prepare from scratch, it takes a larger quantity of the refined product to fill your stomach because these foods do not contain the original food's fiber. Think of crushing a bag of chips versus shredding carrots and celery. The fresh vegetables will satiate your hunger with a smaller volume.

When you eat foods closer to their form at harvest, you will become full with smaller portions. The feeling of fullness stays with you for a longer period too, so you don't need to snack as much. By following this simple lifestyle change, you will eat a smaller quantity of food loaded with vitamins, minerals, fiber, and all the nutrients the human body needs—the way God intended for you to eat.

Pay attention to portion size. Think of your stomach as the size of your fist—before it is stretched out by food. Put less food on your plate than you think you will eat. Use a smaller plate. As soon as you feel full, stop eating and put the timer on for five minutes. When the timer rings, you shouldn't feel hungry anymore since it takes a little while for your brain to recognize your stomach reached its capacity. If you stop eating at the first sign you feel the sensation of fullness, in five minutes your brain receptors catch up with the feeling in your stomach.

Eating Out

Realistically, you won't be able to prepare meals at home all the time. Our lives are busy and many days we are unable to eat at home. Let's first address fast food. Most fast-food restaurants provide a selection of healthy options to choose from, such as a fresh salad with raw ingredients. However, be sure to use either no dressing or as small a portion as you can. If you use more than one fast-food package of salad dressing, you just made your positive eating choice into a negative one. I ask for the salad dressing on the side, and I dip my fork into the dressing before placing food on the fork. That way I get a smaller but flavorful amount of the high-calorie, high-sugar condiment.

Healthy eating choices at a dine-in restaurant are a vegetable plate, fish, or chicken. First, check the menu for the ingredients in your meal choice, and make sure you ask for your food to be served in the healthiest way: no sauces and baked or grilled instead of fried. When your food arrives, the serving size may be substantial. Therefore, when served a large plate of food, before you begin eating, determine how much you will eat to prevent overeating. You might even ask for a to-go container at the beginning of your meal to store what you will not eat at this meal. It is difficult to stop unless you establish boundaries before you begin eating delicious foods.

	Breakfast	Lunch	Snack	Dinner
Food				
Time				
Three Hours Since Last Meal?				
Hungry?				
Feel an Emotion? Describe:				
Satisfied or Stuffed				
Digestive Issue?				
Poor Mental Clarity?				
Bad Mood?				

DAY 33: 80/20 PERCENT RULE

Guide your eating with the 80/20 percent rule. *If you eat healthy 80 percent of the time and not so healthy 20 percent of the time, this will probably be an improvement.* I don't eat perfectly, but with God's help I try. If I mess up, the next day I get to start new, as indicated in:

Because of the LORD's great love we are not consumed,
    for his compassions never fail.
    They are new every morning;
    great is your faithfulness.

Lamentations 3:22–23 (NIV)

Each morning as I wake up, my body tells me how well I ate the previous day. If I did not experience any blood sugar fluctuations, I have a clear mind and abundant energy. The incredible sensation of how God created our bodies to feel motivates me to continue to eat well every day. I am more productive when I eat healthy foods.

However, don't make your expectations too high. Remember the 80/20 rule: if you improve your eating 80 percent of the time, you will improve your diet. This lifestyle change is not an all-or-nothing situation. If you don't follow healthy dietary guidelines 100 percent of the time, don't adopt the belief that you failed. Instead, give yourself grace as God does. Try to do well, but if you don't eat correctly 20 percent of the time, that's okay. It's still probably better than the way you were eating before. Get back on track as soon as you can.

	Breakfast	Lunch	Snack	Dinner
Food				
Time				
Three Hours Since Last Meal?				
Hungry?				
Feel an Emotion? Describe:				
Satisfied or Stuffed				
Digestive Issue?				
Poor Mental Clarity?				
Bad Mood?				

34

DAY 34: JOURNAL TIME

	Breakfast	Lunch	Snack	Dinner
Food				
Time				
Three Hours Since Last Meal?				
Hungry?				
Feel an Emotion? Describe:				
Satisfied or Stuffed				
Digestive Issue?				
Poor Mental Clarity?				
Bad Mood?				

35

DAY 35: SABBATH REFLECTIONS

	Breakfast	Lunch	Snack	Dinner
Food				
Time				
Three Hours Since Last Meal?				
Hungry?				
Feel an Emotion? Describe:				
Satisfied or Stuffed				
Digestive Issue?				
Poor Mental Clarity?				
Bad Mood?				

PART VI
WEEK 6

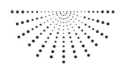

MENU PLAN

WEEKLY MENU PLANNING

When you plan your menu, choose a pleasant spot (outside, by a fire, coffee shop). This may take up to an hour, but is well worth your time and effort. Use the recipes in appendix 4 of *7 Steps to Get Off Sugar and Carbohydrates* (SusanUNeal.com/appendix), another healthy cookbook, or an app on your smartphone to find recipes. I provided a list of healthy food options in appendix 3 to give you ideas of what to cook. Post your menu on the refrigerator, so you know what you planned to cook for each meal during the week.

Cooking from scratch is important. For example, do not buy garlic already minced in a jar. You have no idea how old it is. The nutrients from fruits and vegetables begin to break down as soon as you cut them. Instead, mince a fresh clove of garlic.

It might take longer to cook from scratch, but the food will be more nutritious and low in sugar. Your health is worth it. Your family will appreciate the time you invest into preparing healthy, delicious meals. Make the transition from eating convenience foods, such as processed foods, take out, or eating out, to home cooked food.

Use the following chart to plan out your weekly menu.

Meal	Monday	Tuesday
Breakfast		
Lunch		
Snack		
Dinner		

Meal	Wednesday	Thursday
Breakfast		
Lunch		
Snack		
Dinner		

Meal	Friday	Saturday
Breakfast		
Lunch		
Snack		
Dinner		

Meal	Sunday
Breakfast	
Lunch	
Snack	
Dinner	

WELL-BEING CHART

The following Well-Being Chart will help you determine how habits affect your well-being. Record the number of hours you slept and add a Y for yes and N for no for the other items tracked below. Recognize if there is a correlation between your energy level and mood with the consumption of unhealthy foods. List those foods on the chart.

Your sleep and diet affect your brain. If you slept less than eight hours or ate unhealthy foods, color the box red in the Well-Being Chart. If you experience a day with high energy and clarity of mind color the corresponding boxes green.

Many of the symptoms listed in the Well-Being Chart (energy, brain fog, mood, anxiety, irritability, digestive issues) are affected by the foods you consume.

At the end of the week review your Daily Food Journals and compare it with your Well-Being Chart to determine how you did food wise along with the corresponding symptoms. When you color boxes red (negative symptoms) and green (positive symptoms) it is easier to figure out what type of food makes your body function well and vice-versa. When you find a food culprit, eliminate it from your diet.

Please complete the information below.

Days	36	37	38	39	40	41	42
Hours of Sleep							
Ate Unhealthy Foods: List the foods							
Binged							
Low Energy Level							
Brain Fog							
Bad Mood							
Anxiety							
Irritable							
Digestive Issues							
Physical Activity							
Probiotics							
Spent Time w/ God							

DAY 36: EXERCISE

It doesn't matter what type of exercise you do as long as you do it. Walking, lifting weights, or taking a group fitness class are a few examples of healthy exercise. After you improve your eating habits and begin feeling better, try to exercise for twenty minutes three times a week. Even if you only walk down the road a couple of blocks and come back, start moving.

Record the exercise you perform in the Fitness Tracker chart in this journal. If you haven't been exercising, determine why. Is it because you don't have the time? Or are you too tired?

_____

Is there a type of physical endeavor you enjoyed when you were younger? Maybe it's time to try it again. I enjoyed swimming as a child, so I try to swim laps in my pool a couple of times a week. Figure out what you like to do and put it on your calendar. Ask a family member, friend, neighbor, or even your accountability partner to join you on a regular basis, so you can encourage each other to keep up this beneficial habit.

Exercise is a positive coping strategy for dealing with stress; it burns off adrenaline and improves sleep. Do you engage in relaxation techniques such as Christian yoga or meditation? Yoga eases pain, improves depression, and boosts metabolism and immunity. Yoga and meditation calm the mind and body. I created several Christian yoga products including DVDs, books, and card decks available at Christianyoga.com.

Do you routinely exercise? If yes, what type of activity do you perform? Do you enjoy this type of exercise?

_____

If you do not routinely exercise, what type of workout do you enjoy?

_____

How can you incorporate an enjoyable form of activity into your life?

_____

_____

	Breakfast	Lunch	Snack	Dinner
Food				
Time				
Three Hours Since Last Meal?				
Hungry?				
Feel an Emotion? Describe:				
Satisfied or Stuffed				
Digestive Issue?				
Poor Mental Clarity?				
Bad Mood?				

37

DAY 37: PRACTICE GRATITUDE

When you embrace a mind-set of gratitude, dopamine releases in your brain. Remember that dopamine, the feel-good neurohormone, releases when you eat sugar and wheat. Instead of getting the positive feeling from a bad habit, get it from a good one—by journaling gratefulness. Next time you want to eat something unhealthy, grab this journal instead and record what you are grateful for in the Gratitude Log at the beginning of this book.

To get an into an attitude of gratitude, I listen to praise music, whether I am cooking, driving, or getting ready for work. Listening to worship music gets me into the mood to praise God. That's when dopamine releases and I feel the Holy Spirit's vibrancy within me. Fill your mind, heart, and body with the Spirit of God by putting the right things in your spirit.

Fix your thoughts on what is true and good and right. Think about things that are pure and lovely, and dwell on the fine, good things in others. Think about all you can praise God for and be glad about.

Philippians 4:8 (TLB)

Lord,

I want to focus my thoughts on "what is true and good and right," not on negative things. Help me to change my mind-set and priorities so I focus on the things that are important to you. Thank you for giving me gladness when I praise you! Jesus, through your name I pray. Amen.

Journal about what you are grateful for:

_____

_____

_____

_____

_____

_____

_____

	Breakfast	Lunch	Snack	Dinner
Food				
Time				
Three Hours Since Last Meal?				
Hungry?				
Feel an Emotion? Describe:				
Satisfied or Stuffed				
Digestive Issue?				
Poor Mental Clarity?				
Bad Mood?				

38

DAY 38: FRUIT OF THE SPIRIT: SELF-CONTROL

Another reason some people struggle to eat healthy foods is their bodies betray their mental commitment. It may not be just a matter of self-control; you may have a food addiction (day 9) or overgrowth of Candida (day 10) in the GI tract that causes you to overeat. There could also be an emotional connection to food (day 22). Finding out the root issue is instrumental to being freed from the compulsion to overeat.

We need to recognize how addictions affect us physically, so we can be prepared with the mental ammunition needed to stay strong. Food addiction is quite prevalent in our society today. It is a biochemical disorder that cannot be controlled through self-control. An addiction causes a person to repeat the same type of behavior despite life-damaging consequences. That is why we need to learn to use God's spiritual weapons.

Have you ever relied on self-control to overcome temptations of the flesh but failed? We need to use God's power to conquer temptations and food issues. How do we access his power? Let's look for the answer in the Bible. Speak these verses out loud:

. . .

In your hands are strength and power
to exalt and give strength to all.

1 Chronicles 29:12 (NIV)

You are their glorious strength.
It pleases you to make us strong.

Psalm 89:17

From these verses, we see that "the Lord" can "give strength to all" and it pleases him "to make us strong." The transformation from food addiction cannot come from dietary boundaries and self-control alone; it must come from God helping you. Turn to the Lord when you want to eat inappropriately. Explore your emotions with him and ask him to stabilize your feelings. Allow him to minister to your heart and mind, and your eating habits will improve.

Have you tried to overcome inappropriate eating before? If you failed, you were probably dealing with the issue through your own resolve. Instead, call on the power of the Holy Spirit to change you from the inside out. With God's help, you can overcome and succeed.

The LORD hears his people when they call to him for help.
He rescues them from all their troubles.
The LORD is close to the brokenhearted;
he rescues those whose spirits are crushed.
The righteous person faces many troubles,
but the LORD comes to the rescue each time.

Psalm 34:17–19

Ask God to help you overcome your struggle with food.

_____

_____

_____

Psalm 89:17 states that it pleases God to make us strong. So ask him to give you his supernatural strength to make healthy eating choices and not fall prey to temptations.

_____

_____

_____

Lord,

I know you hear me when I call for help, so I am asking you to rescue me from my struggles with food. Strengthen me each time I am tempted. Please help me to remember to always call upon you. Thank you. In Jesus's name, I pray. Amen.

	Breakfast	Lunch	Snack	Dinner
Food				
Time				
Three Hours Since Last Meal?				
Hungry?				
Feel an Emotion? Describe:				
Satisfied or Stuffed				
Digestive Issue?				
Poor Mental Clarity?				
Bad Mood?				

39

DAY 39: PLAN FOR THE PITFALLS

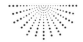

No one is perfect. You will have days when you eat sugar, wheat, or processed foods. That's okay. This happens to everyone; don't let it discourage you. Share your feelings with your accountability/prayer partner. Pray together. Please join my closed Facebook group, 7 Steps to Get Off Sugar, Carbs, and Gluten and share with me how you are doing. If you would like healthy living tips please like my Facebook page at Facebook.com/HealthyLivingSeries/.

Changing the way you eat will be a challenging task, but one you can conquer. If you relapse, get up, brush the dust off yourself, and start again. Realize what triggered your cravings. Was it your emotions? Did you write about your feelings, obstacles, and victories in the sixth and seventh days of this journal? These pages were left blank for that purpose.

Did you complete your Daily Food Journal and record when you overate in the Binge Eating Tracker? Have you figured out what triggered you to overeat, and what you might do the next time you are tempted by recording it in the Temptation/Struggle Log? Through journaling you can identify your triggers and strategize how to avoid them. By now you should be well on your way to figuring out your health puzzle.

It is normal for people to stay the course and then fall off the wagon and binge. This cycle continues to repeat itself, but as you continue to turn to God and rely on his strength, slowly but surely you will gain control of your body, mind, and spirit. The changes in your eating habits are a lifelong lifestyle journey so you can live the abundant life Jesus wants you to experience. Not a life filled with disease and unwanted, unhealthy symptoms.

If you did not track everything in this journal but still want to make further improvements in your health and weight, go back and fill in the charts. If you do you will get positive results.

Make check marks by the charts you completed in this journal:
    Gratitude Log
    Victory Log
    Temptation/Struggle Log
    Binge Eating Tracker
    Issue Tracker
    New Healthy Living Habits Log
    Water Tracker
    Steps Tracker
    Fitness Tracker
    Well-Being Chart
    Daily Food Journal
    Appendix 2: My Battle Strategies Plan

I am proud of you for your effort. May God bless your endeavor to improve your health and well-being.

	Breakfast	Lunch	Snack	Dinner
Food				
Time				
Three Hours Since Last Meal?				
Hungry?				
Feel an Emotion? Describe:				
Satisfied or Stuffed				
Digestive Issue?				
Poor Mental Clarity?				
Bad Mood?				

40

DAY 40: IMPROVE YOUR HEALTH

After six weeks I hope you feel like a new person. Hopefully some bothersome symptoms have already disappeared, as well as some excess weight. Maybe big chores, like house cleaning, don't seem so difficult anymore, or perhaps you feel like putting on a cute outfit and attending a social event. As you continue to nourish your body, weak-functioning cells will be replaced by new ones, and your body will work to heal itself of diseases the way the Lord intended.

As a certified health and wellness coach, I encourage and guide others to regain their health. A client told me her pediatric endocrinologist diagnosed her son as obese and prediabetic. We reviewed the types of food her family ate and developed a plan to cut out unhealthy foods. She resolved to eliminate wheat, milk, and fruit juice from her family's diet. I encouraged her to try to improve their eating habits 80 percent of the time and not worry about what they ate the other 20 percent of the time, since no one can be perfect. If you would like me to assist you on this journey to improve your health as your wellness coach go to SusanUNeal.com/Health-Coaching. May God bless your endeavor to improve your health.

. . .

Dear friend, I hope all is well with you and that you are as healthy in body as you are strong in spirit.

3 John 2

Lord,

It is my greatest desire that this journal strengthened my fellow brothers and sisters in Christ. Please help the reader to put the health puzzle together so he or she may experience the abundant life you designed. Bless all those who read this journal.

Thank you. In Jesus's name, I pray. Amen.

	Breakfast	Lunch	Snack	Dinner
Food				
Time				
Three Hours Since Last Meal?				
Hungry?				
Feel an Emotion? Describe:				
Satisfied or Stuffed				
Digestive Issue?				
Poor Mental Clarity?				
Bad Mood?				

41

DAY 41: JOURNAL TIME

	Breakfast	Lunch	Snack	Dinner
Food				
Time				
Three Hours Since Last Meal?				
Hungry?				
Feel an Emotion? Describe:				
Satisfied or Stuffed				
Digestive Issue?				
Poor Mental Clarity?				
Bad Mood?				

42

DAY 42: SABBATH REFLECTIONS

	Breakfast	Lunch	Snack	Dinner
Food				
Time				
Three Hours Since Last Meal?				
Hungry?				
Feel an Emotion? Describe:				
Satisfied or Stuffed				
Digestive Issue?				
Poor Mental Clarity?				
Bad Mood?				

APPENDIX 1: FOOD ADDICTION
BATTLE STRATEGIES

1. Complete the logs, charts, and journaling sections of this book.
2. Ask a friend to be your accountability and prayer partner.
3. Find a specific Bible verse to oppose your food issue, write it on an index card, and memorize it. Speak the verse out loud every time you feel the urge to eat unhealthy foods.
4. Determine food triggers by writing them down in the Temptation/Struggle Log and avoid the trigger.
5. Record every time you overeat in the Binge Eating Tracker.
6. When you are tempted to overeat or eat unhealthy food:

- pray
- go for a walk
- recite your Bible verse
- call your prayer partner
- drink two glasses of water
- listen to praise music and worship God
- spend time with and meditate about God
- write in this journal

7. When you eat any unhealthy food, be sure to journal afterward— every single time. Figure out what you told yourself that validated why it was okay to eat the item. Then go through the Five Spiritual Steps to Freedom from Addiction. If you journal and implement this five-step plan every time you binge, you will experience success. This is part of retraining your mind.

8. Implement the Five Spiritual Steps to Freedom from Addiction:

- Name what controls you.
- Submit yourself completely to God.
- Use the name of Jesus.
- Use the Word of God.
- Praise God and practice gratitude.

Complete the study *Christian Study Guide for 7 Steps to Get Off Sugar and Carbohydrates.*

APPENDIX 2: MY BATTLE STRATEGIES PLAN

1.

2.

3.

4.

5.

6.

7.

8.

9.

10.

APPENDIX 3: HEALTHY FOOD OPTIONS

The following daily meal categories include a list of appropriate healthy food options for your menu planning and shopping lists.

Breakfast

- oatmeal with pecans and cinnamon
- pancakes made with almond flour (recipe link: Pinterest.com/SusanUNeal/breakfast/)
- quinoa with a smashed banana, almond milk, and walnuts
- scrambled eggs with hash browns
- omelet with green onions, red peppers, and mushrooms
- berries with plain Greek yogurt
- chia parfait with fruit
- homemade granola with berries and/or Greek yogurt
- hash browns with onions, peppers, and a sliced avocado on top
- mashed avocado with two fried eggs on top
- pancakes made with two eggs and one smashed banana

Lunch

- a salad or vegetable plate, if eating out
- romaine lettuce wrap sandwich with any meat or vegetable
- cucumber sandwich—cut a cucumber in half and load it with meat (not processed packaged lunch meat) and veggies
- salad with fish, chicken, nuts, or avocado
- baked potato bar with olive oil, broccoli, scallions, and sunflower seeds
- guacamole or hummus with sliced vegetables
- whole avocado and an heirloom tomato
- baked sweet potato with butter, cinnamon, and honey

Snack

- sliced green apple with almond or cashew butter
- berries with whipped cream made with coconut milk
- raw vegetables with hummus or guacamole
- boiled egg or deviled eggs (made with organic mayonnaise)
- carrots and celery sticks
- berries with slivered almonds
- nuts—raw almonds, pecans, pistachios, macadamia nuts, or cashews
- organic popcorn popped on the stove (not microwave popcorn)

Dinner

- chicken fajitas with guacamole, lettuce, tomato, and avocado on a coconut tortilla wrap (available at health food stores)
- spaghetti with a baked spaghetti squash for the noodles
- steak, mushrooms, green beans with slivered almonds, and a salad
- salmon, sautéed red cabbage, and wild rice
- baked or grilled chicken, quinoa, and sautéed or grilled zucchini and yellow squash

- chili made with lean meat
- fish, salad, and asparagus
- beef stew with potato, carrots, celery, bok choy, and onions
- black bean soup
- fresh field peas with sliced tomatoes, fried okra, and corn pone bread (recipe in appendix 4 of *7 Steps to Get Off Sugar and Carbohydrates*. You can obtain a printable version of this appendix at SusanUNeal.com/appendix).
- shrimp fettuccine alfredo with shirataki noodles, and a salad
- roasted whole chicken with onions, potatoes, carrots, and bok choy
- salad with berries, nuts, and seeds

Dessert

- dark chocolate (at least 70 percent chocolate)
- dark chocolate almond cookies (recipe in appendix 4 of *7 Steps to Get Off Sugar and Carbohydrates*)
- chocolate nut clusters
- dark chocolate–covered strawberries
- one dried date to seven pecan halves (be careful, as dates are high in sugar)

NOTES

Well-Being Chart
1. Dale E. Bredesen, Edwin C. Amos, Jonathan Canick, Mary Ackerley, Cyrus Raji, Milan Fiala, and Jamila Ahdidan, "Reversal of cognitive decline in Alzheimer's disease," *Aging*, June 2016.

Daily Food Journal
2. Ibid.

Day 3: Healthy Eating Guidelines
3. John Brennan, "What is Roundup Ready Corn," Sciencing, April 25, 2017

Day 10: Candida
4. "Candida Yeast Infection, Leaky Gut, Irritable Bowel and Food Allergies," National Candida Center, https://www.nationalcandida-center.com/Leaky-Gut-and-Candida-Yeast-Infection-s/1823.htm.

Day 12: Foods to Eliminate
5. Stacy Simon, "World Health Organization Says Processed Meat Causes Cancer," *American Cancer Society*, October 26, 2015,

https://www.cancer.org/latest-news/world-health-organization-says-processed-meat-causes-cancer.html.

Day 19: Five Spiritual Steps to Freedom from Addiction

6. Larry Lea, *The Weapons of Your Warfare: Equipping Yourself to Defeat the Enemy* (Reading: Cox and Wyman, Ltd. 1990), 126, 182.

ABOUT THE AUTHOR

Susan U. Neal, RN, MBA, MHS, is an award-winning author, speaker, and certified health and wellness coach whose background in nursing and health services led her to seek new ways to educate and coach people to overcome health challenges. She published the award-winning book *7 Steps to Get Off Sugar and Carbohydrates* and its corresponding Bible study *Christian Study Guide for 7 Steps to Get Off Sugar and Carbohydrates*. Her other books include, *Solving the Gluten Puzzle*, *Scripture Yoga*, a #1 Amazon best-seller, and *Yoga for Beginners*. Her passion and mission is to help others improve their health and weight. To learn more about Susan visit her website at SusanUNeal.com.

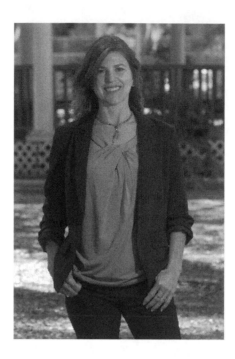

Susan has been interviewed on the *Bridges Show* on Christian Television Network (CTN), Moody Radio, Blog Talk Radio, and Premier Christian Radio from the UK.

Susan founded Scripture Yoga™, a form of Christian yoga, and enjoys leading classes at her church and fitness club. She is a speaker and enjoys teaching Scripture Yoga™ sessions at women's retreats, Christian conferences, and yoga retreats.

Previously Susan worked as a kidney transplant nurse at Shands Hospital in Gainesville, Florida; assistant administrator at Mayo Clinic Jacksonville; and quality assurance nurse at Blue Cross Blue Shield of Florida. Currently, she owns her own business, Christian Yoga, LLC, and publishes Christian products, along with teaching group fitness classes.

Connect with Susan Online

Susan created the Healthy Living Series blog to provide healthy lifestyle tips and the latest scientific findings regarding foods and health. She also posts menu and grocery shopping list to help with planning healthy menus. You can subscribe to the blog at Susan-UNeal.com/healthy-living-blog.

You can follow Susan on:
    Facebook.com/SusanUllrichNeal
    Facebook.com/ScriptureYoga/
    Facebook.com/HealthyLivingSeries/
    Twitter.com/SusanNealYoga
    Youtube.com/c/SusanNealScriptureYoga/
    Pinterest.com/SusanUNeal/
    Instagram.com/healthylivingseries/
    Linkedin.com/in/susannealyoga/

Follow Susan on BookBub to get an email when she releases a new book or her books go on sale at BookBub.com/authors/susan-u-neal.

SusanUNeal.com and ChristianYoga.com
SusanNeal@bellsouth.net

OTHER PRODUCTS BY SUSAN NEAL

HEALTHY LIVING SERIES COURSE & BOOKS

7 Steps to Reclaim Your Health and Optimal Weight Online Course

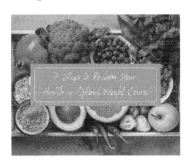

If you need additional support making this lifestyle change, purchase my course, 7 Steps to Reclaim Your Health and Optimal Weight at Susan-UNeal.com/courses/7-steps-to-get-off-sugar-and-carbs-course. In this course I walk you through all the material covered in my Healthy Living Series.

I teach you the root causes of inappropriate eating habits and help you resolve those issues. One solved, taming your appetite is much easier. Learn how to change your eating habits successfully once and for all.

Book 1: *7 Steps to Get Off Sugar and Carbohydrates*

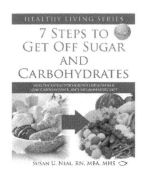

Over half of Americans live with a chronic illness and forty percent suffer from obesity, primarily due to the overconsumption of sugar and refined carbohydrates. *Seven Steps to Get Off Sugar and Carbohydrates* provides a day-by-day plan to wean your body off these addictive products and regain your health. These changes in your eating habits will start your lifestyle journey to the abundant life Jesus wants you to experience, not a life filled with disease and poor health.

You will learn how to:

- eliminate brain fog, cure diseases, and lose weight
- choose foods that benefit versus foods that damage—the ones God gave us to eat, not the food industry
- find healthy food alternatives and plan your menu
- recognize the emotional reasons we overeat and the science behind food addiction and a candida infection (overgrowth of yeast in the gut)
- identify food triggers and use God's Word to fight impulsive eating
- locate resources—educational videos and books, meal planning, support organizations, and recipes.

Jesus said in John 10:10, "The thief's purpose is to steal, kill and destroy. My purpose is to give life in all its fullness" (TLB). Are you living life in its fullness? Is your health or weight impeding you from embracing a healthy, bountiful life? If you take these simple seven steps, you will regain the life God created you for. You will love the new you! To purchase go to ChristianYoga.com/yoga-books-decks.

Christian Study Guide for 7 Steps to Get Off Sugar and Carbohydrates

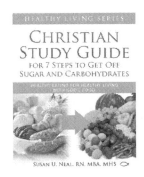

CHRISTIAN STUDY GUIDE
FOR 7 STEPS TO GET OFF
SUGAR AND CARBOHYDRATES

SUSAN U. NEAL, RN, MBA, MHS

More than half of Americans suffer with a chronic disease and 40 percent are obese. Struggling with health problems is not our true destiny. Jesus promised us a life of abundance. He also told us, "The thief's purpose is to steal, kill, and destroy" (John 10:10 TLB). Shortening our lifespan through our unhealthy food patterns is the enemy's perfect scheme.

Many of the health problems we suffer are connected to eating habits. Change your life by changing the types of food you eat. Learn which foods are beneficial and which foods make you sick. Don't struggle on your own to make necessary lifestyle changes. Learn how to mobilize God's power. Through the Holy Spirit, you become strong and able to accomplish what you cannot achieve by your own efforts. When you apply God's wisdom, along with accurate knowledge about today's food, you will improve your health and weight and defeat the enemy.

This study guide provides a group experience to help implement the plans in *7 Steps to Get Off Sugar and Carbohydrates*. Accountability and encouragement improve your chance for success as you learn to become a healthy steward of the resources you've been given. You only have one body, and you want it to carry you through this life gracefully. Reclaim the abundant life God wants you to live. Take this journey to recover your health and achieve all the blessings the Lord has in store for you.

Healthy Living Series: 3 Books in 1: 7 Steps to Get Off Sugar and Carbohydrates; Christian Study Guide for 7 Steps to Get Off Sugar and Carbohydrates; Healthy Living Journal

This mega book contains all three of the Healthy Living Series books:

7 Steps to Get Off Sugar and Carbohydrates
Christian Study Guide for 7 Steps to Get Off Sugar and Carbohydrates
Healthy Living Journal.

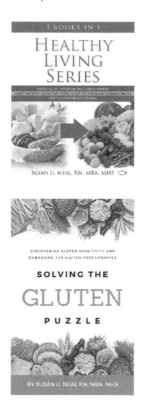

Solving the Gluten Puzzle

Are you experiencing symptoms that you or your doctor don't understand? Ruling out a gluten-related diagnosis may move you one step closer to wellness. Discovering whether you have celiac disease, gluten sensitivity, wheat sensitivity, or a wheat allergy is like piecing together a puzzle. Random pieces don't make sense and won't until the whole picture fits together. *Solving the Gluten Puzzle* explains the symptoms, diagnostic tests, and treatment for these ailments.

Nearly 10 percent of the population is affected by one of four gluten-related disorders, which can cause more than two hundred symptoms, most of which are not digestive. These disorders can strike at any age. Unfortunately, a single diagnostic test to determine gluten sensitivity does not exist. Consequently, up to 80 percent of individuals go undiagnosed. Determine whether you suffer from one of these conditions and how to cure your symptoms by embracing a gluten-free lifestyle.

HOW TO PREVENT, IMPROVE, AND REVERSE ALZHEIMER'S AND DEMENTIA

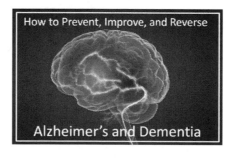

This pamphlet provides twenty-four interventions you can do to prevent, improve, or even reverse Alzheimer's and dementia. There is finally hope. To order this pamphlet go to SusanUNeal.com/appendix.

YOGA BOOKS

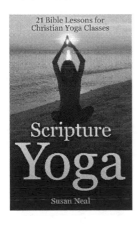

Scripture Yoga assists yoga students in creating a Christian atmosphere for their classes. Choose from twenty-one lessons, each a mini–Bible study that will deepen the participants' walk with God.

Each lesson contains a scriptural theme designed to facilitate meditation on God's Word. The Scripture verses are arranged progressively to facilitate an understanding of each Bible study topic. The Bible lessons will enhance the spiritual depth of your yoga class and make it appropriate and desirable for Christian participants.

Check your poses with photographs of over sixty yoga postures taken on the sugar-white sands of the Emerald Coast of Florida. A detailed description of each pose is provided with full-page photographs so postures are easily seen and replicated. You can purchase these books at ChristianYoga.com/yoga-books-decks.

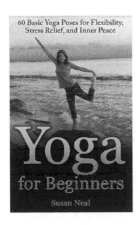

Yoga for Beginners eases you into the inner peace you long for at an easy, step-by-step beginner's pace. Through Susan's gentle encouragement, you will learn how to improve your flexibility and relieve stress. A broad range of yoga poses provides many options for the beginner- to intermediate-level student.

In *Yoga for Beginners* you get it more than basic yoga postures. You will begin to breathe a new sense of well-being when you follow Susan's life-changing eating practices. Learn not only what to eat but also why. This book includes:

1. Sixty basic yoga poses with full-page photographs and detailed explanations
2. Three different routines to give variety
3. Warm-up stretches
4. Injury prevention and posture modification suggestions
5. How to ease pain and anxiety
6. Essential components of yoga such as breathing and stretching
7. Meditation techniques to reduce stress
8. Low-glycemic diet guidelines to obtain optimal weight
9. Causes of sugar cravings and solutions for controlling them

CHRISTIAN YOGA CARD DECKS

Scripture Yoga Card Decks include a yoga pose on one side and a theme-based Bible verse on the other. The decks assist Christian yoga instructors and students in creating a Christian atmosphere for their classes through meditating on the Word of God. You can order the card decks at ChristianYoga.com/yoga-books-decks.

The Fruit of the Spirit Deck

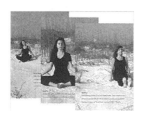
This lesson, The Fruit of the Spirit, describes each of the fruits of the spirit including love, joy, peace, patience, kindness, goodness, gentleness, faithfulness, and self-control. It is a mini– Bible study that will deepen the participants' walk with God.

The Scripture verses are arranged progressively to facilitate a complete understanding of the Bible study topic. The Bible lesson will enhance the spiritual depth of your yoga class, and make it appropriate and desirable for Christian participants.

How to Receive God's Peace Deck

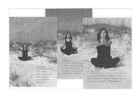

This lesson, How to Receive God's Peace, walks the participant through the steps needed to cast fear and anxiety on God and receive his peace. It is a peace the world cannot give. This mini–Bible study will deepen the participants' walk with God.

SCRIPTURE YOGA DVDS

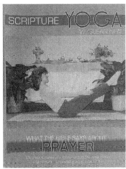

What The Bible Says about Prayer

In this session we explore different aspects of prayer. We look at the "when, where, and how" of prayer illustrated through Bible verses and stories. In this DVD, I share with you many facets of prayer. Prayer is more powerful than we can imagine. This DVD will help your prayer life. To purchase go to Christianyoga.com/dvd-products.

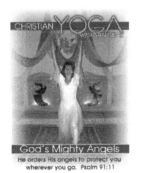

God's Mighty Angels Christian Yoga DVD

Enter the realm of God's mighty angels and find out how they intercede in our lives. Angels are God's messengers and he sends them to protect you wherever you go (Psalm 91:11). Over twenty verses about angels are recited during the class. This is a gentle yoga class that includes twenty-five minutes of stretching and fifty-five minutes of yoga postures for an eighty-minute class. To purchase go to ChristianYoga.com/dvd-products.

Manufactured by Amazon.ca
Bolton, ON

19154120R00136